MANAGING CANCER

MANAGING CANCER

The African-American's Guide to Prevention, Diagnosis, and Treatment

REVISED AND UPDATED

George H. Rawls, M.D., F.A.C.S.
Frank P. Lloyd, Jr., M.D., F.A.C.S.
Michael T. Slaughter, M.D., Ph.D.

AND HERBERT STERN, PH.D.

FOREWORD BY
LaSALLE D. LEFFELL, JR., M.D., F.A.C.S.

HILTON PUBLISHING COMPANY • CHICAGO, ILLINOIS

© 2002, 2006 by Hilton Publishing Company, Munster, IN

Hilton Publishing Company
Chicago, IL

Direct all correspondence to:
Hilton Publishing Company
1630 45th Street, Suite 103
Munster, IN 46321
219-922-4868
www.hiltonpub.com

ISBN: 0-9764443-2-1

Publisher's Cataloging-in-Publication

Rawls, George H.
    Managing cancer : the African-American's guide to prevention, diagnosis, and treatment / George H. Rawls, Frank P. Lloyd, Jr., Michael T. Slaughter, and Herbert Stern. — 2nd ed.
        p. cm.
    Includes bibliographical references and index.
    ISBN: 0-9764443-2-1

    1. Cancer—Popular works. 2. African Americans—Health and Hygiene. I. Lloyd, Frank P. II. Slaughter, Michael T. III. Stern, Herbert. III. Title.

RC282.B55R39 2001   616.99'4'008996073
                                      QBI01–200159

Printed and bound in the United States of America

*This book is dedicated by
Frank P. Lloyd, Jr., Michael T. Slaughter,
and George H. Rawls to the many cancer
patients they have treated and managed.*

CONTENTS

PART III *Human Questions*

FOREWORD

LaSalle D. Leffall, Jr., M.D., F.A.C.S.
Charles R. Drew Professor of Surgery,
Howard University College of Medicine;
Former President, American Cancer Society;
Former President, American College of Surgeons

THIS WELL-WRITTEN, thoroughly researched book contains valuable information about African Americans and cancer. The authors have compiled facts that, if heeded, can lead to better health. Appropriate attention is given to prevention, screening, diagnosis, treatment, and rehabilitation. Further, the roles of spirituality and faith are not neglected but rather emphasized, whatever one's religious beliefs.

Recognizing that African Americans have the highest incidence of common cancers such as lung, prostate, and colorectal, the authors state clearly what can be done to achieve earlier diagnosis and thus better cure rates.

What gives this book a special touch are the personal stories involving patients, the senior author himself, and his family. Many of these stories are poignant, revealing examples of individual courage as testimony to the endurance, if not the triumph, of the human spirit in crisis. Particularly appealing is how passion, hope, and sensitivity as essential elements of patient care are interwoven throughout the book.

The senior author, George H. Rawls, a highly respected surgeon with a wealth of clinical experience, has brought his vast talents to this book, making it an even more prized possession for those interested in knowing more about cancer. I enthusiastically recommend this book for the lay public. Following the advice in it can help save lives.

ACKNOWLEDGMENTS

THE AUTHORS ACKNOWLEDGE with gratitude the excellent assistance of Judie Aitken and Karen Spear, Ph.D., of the Methodist Research Institute, Methodist Hospital, Indianapolis, for typing, reviewing, and providing helpful suggestions. Betty Johnson of the National Cancer Institute helped immeasurably by providing SEER information, monograms, and illustrations. Anthony Saffioti of the American Cancer Society and Lippincott Williams and Wilkins graciously granted us permission to use information from *CA: A Cancer Journal for Clinicians*. Finally, thanks to Nicky Wooden for his editorial suggestion, and to Vry Corscaden for telling us about her experiences with imaging and the macrobiotic diet.

PART I

Knowledge Not of Fear

ONE

Cancer and Blacks

TO LEARN THAT A CLOSE relative has cancer can be devastating. I know. Not long ago, an aunt who is dear to me died of colon cancer. My mother died from ovarian cancer, and my brother died from complications that followed prostate surgery.

To learn that one has cancer oneself can also be a terrible experience. I know. I have been treated for thyroid cancer, and recently, I learned that I may now have prostate cancer.

Perhaps more than any other disease, cancer breeds anxiety. Even after the doctor has declared one cured, many fears can linger. I know those fears also:

- Did the surgeon leave behind a few malignant cells that may become active in the future?
- Might the cancer return?
- Will I ever be completely cured so my fears can come to an end.

Yes, I know these fears, but I also know that with the right effort of heart and will, they too can be managed.

3

CANCER AND BLACKS

Cancer is particularly hard on black people. The overall incidence of cancer in African Americans is 512.3 per 100,000, while in whites it is 479.7. A similarly disturbing disparity holds true of mortality rates: in African Americans, 339.4 per 100,000 men, and in whites, 242.3 per 100,000. For women, the numbers were 194.3 for black women versus 164.5 for white women. As if that weren't bad enough, from the early 1960s to 2000, the mortality rates for black men rose 62 percent and for black women 16 percent, compared to 19 percent for men and 5 percent for women of all races combined. By 1992, the age-adjusted mortality rates were 32 percent higher for blacks than for all races combined.

There has been some improvement, but the rate of incidence is still far too high.

These are hard statistics, hard enough to lead some researchers to call these terrible increases the most significant health crisis of the twentieth century. The mortality rates for nearly every cancer—stomach cancer is the exception—are higher for blacks than are the rates among white cancer patients.

For the time being, we can only speculate about why the death rate from cancer is so high among us. Here are some of the stronger theories:

- Poor screening and educational programs
- Diagnosis in blacks occurs at more advanced stages of cancer, when treatments are less likely to be effective
- Increased environmental risks, especially among poor people, where exposure to asbestos and other toxic materials is likely to be higher, and where high incidence of cigarette smoking, along with bad diet, increases these risks
- Lack of access to caring health institutions
- Lack of insurance

TABLE 1

AFRICAN AMERICAN TO WHITE CANCER MORTALITY RATE* RATIOS, US, 1997–2001

MALES

CANCER	AFRICAN AMERICAN RATE	WHITE RATE	AFRICAN AMERICAN/ WHITE RATIO
Prostate	70.4	28.8	2.4
Larynx	5.4	2.3	2.3
Stomach	13.3	5.8	2.3
Myeloma	9.0	4.4	2.0
Oral cavity and pharynx	7.5	3.9	1.9
Esophagus	11.7	7.4	1.6
Liver and intrahepatic bile duct	9.3	6.1	1.5
Small intestine	0.7	0.5	1.4
Colon and rectum	34.3	24.8	1.4
Lung and bronchus	104.1	76.6	1.4
Pancreas	15.0	12.0	1.3
Kidney and renal pelvis	5.3	6.2	1.0
Hodgkin lymphoma	0.6	0.6	1.0
Leukemia	9.0	10.5	0.9
Thyroid	0.4	0.5	0.8
Urinary bladder	5.6	7.9	0.7
Non-Hodgkin lymphoma	7.4	10.8	0.7
Brain and other nervous system	3.3	6.0	0.5
Melanoma of the skin	0.5	4.4	0.1
All malignant neoplasms	352.2	250.5	1.4

FEMALES

CANCER	AFRICAN AMERICAN RATE	WHITE RATE	AFRICAN AMERICAN/ WHITE RATIO
Myeloma	6.6	2.9	2.3
Stomach	6.3	2.8	2.3
Uterine cervix	5.5	2.6	2.2
Esophagus	3.2	1.7	1.9
Larynx	0.9	0.5	1.8
Uterine corpus	6.9	3.9	1.8
Pancreas	12.8	8.9	1.4
Colon and rectum	24.5	17.1	1.4
Liver and intrahepatic bile duct	3.8	2.7	1.4
Breast	35.4	26.4	1.3
Urinary bladder	2.9	2.3	1.3
Oral Cavity and pharynx	2.0	1.6	1.3
Ovary	9.2	7.5	1.2
Kidney and renal pelvis	2.7	2.8	1.0
Non-Hodgkin lymphoma	39.9	41.6	1.0
Leukemia	5.4	6.0	0.9
Brain and other nervous system	4.6	7.2	0.6
Melanoma of the skin	0.5	2.0	0.3
All malignant neoplasms	200.4	169.1	1.2

* Rates are per 100,000 and age-adjusted to the 2000 US population standard. † Site selected if deaths greater than 50.
Source: National Center for Health Statistics, Centers for Disease Control and Prevention

FIGURE 1

SEER INCIDENCE, 1992-2002

Breast, Lung/Brochus, and Colorectal Cancers, for Females by Race/Ethnicity

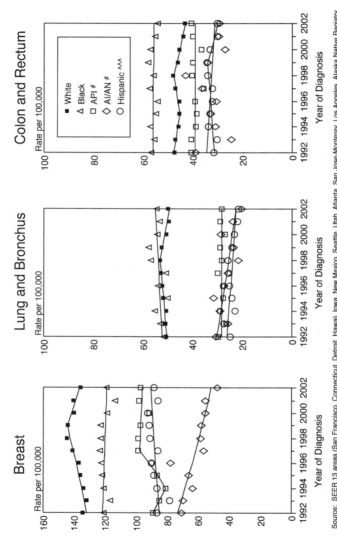

Source: SEER 13 areas (San Francisco, Connecticut, Detroit, Hawaii, Iowa, New Mexico, Seattle, Utah, Atlanta, San Jose-Monterey, Los Angeles, Alaska Native Registry and Rural Georgia). Incidence data for Hispanics excludes cases from Detroit, Hawaii, Alaska Native Registry and Rural Georgia.
Rates are age-adjusted to the 2000 US Std Population (19 age groups - Census P25-1103).
Regression lines are calculated using the Joinpoint Regression Program Version 3.0, April 2005, National Cancer Institute.
API = Asian/Pacific Islander. AI/AN = American Indian/Alaska Native.
^^^ Hispanic is not mutually exclusive from Whites, Blacks, Asian/Pacific Islanders, and American Indians/Alaska Natives.

Surveillance, Epidemiology, and End Results (SEER) Program (www.seer.cancer.gov) SEER*Stat Database: Incidence - SEER 9 Regs Public-Use, Nov 2004 Sub (1973-2002), National Cancer Institute, DCCPS, Surveillance Research Program, Cancer Statistics Branch, released April 2005, based on the November 2004 submission.

- Health care providers not offering current best treatment therapies to minority patients.

One reason blacks may be diagnosed for cancer later than whites is poverty. We all know the numbers. According to Census Bureau figure for 2004, the median income for all races was $44,389; for whites it was $46,697, and for African Americans it was $30,134. In 2004, the poverty rate for whites was 8.6%, for Hispanics, 21%, and for blacks, 24.7%. Think about it: roughly a quarter of our people live in poverty!

Naturally, the health implications of such statistics are devastating. Harold Freeman, former president of the American Cancer Society, observes that, because of poverty, many blacks must concern themselves with day-to-day survival priorities such as food, shelter, and avoidance of crime, and don't have much heart left over to care for their health.

One reason blacks may be diagnosed for cancer later than whites is poverty.

Even when poor people *do* attempt to care for their health, they are likely to have bad experiences. A poor person suffering from cancer symptoms will probably go first to the emergency room, and may then be referred to a clinic. If the person fails to follow through by going to the clinic, or if he or she is discouraged by the long lines or, perhaps, by the fear of learning that he or she is ill, the diagnosis may be delayed until the condition is no longer curable.

Poverty may also account for an often fatalistic attitude toward cancer among blacks, and for lack of the knowledge that would guarantee prompt and effective treatment. In our own practices, we've treated black women with breast cancer brought in against their wills by family members; "I thought that it was hopeless," these women often remark.

Although the symptoms suffered by these women were sometimes terrible prognosis was often good. The tumors, in many cases, had spread locally but not throughout the body. That's why early diagnosis is so important: it gives us a chance to catch such tumors *before* they spread outside the breast.

Fatalism can take another form. I've had patients come to me announcing, "I know I have cancer. Take it out." Often tests would show clearly that the problem was mastitis, which, though painful and, like cancer, produces lumps, is a minor ailment and easily treatable. Only with the greatest difficulty could I assure these patients that they did not have cancer. Fear can distort reality in any number of ways.

From a doctor's point of view, sensitive and compassionate care is essential to the treatment of black men and women. But patients must take on responsibility, too. Their job is to become health activists, people who understand their bodies are their responsibility, in sickness as in health.

Patients must take on responsibility.

The cancer patient's attitude and knowledge increase or decrease his or her risk. Often it is ignorance that causes people to delay seeking treatment promptly or to refuse treatment altogether, and knowledge that causes them to seek out diagnosis and treatment early enough for these to lead to cure.

Fear itself, we've seen, is sometimes grounded in ignorance. But it may be grounded in realism as well. People may fear that the costs of surgery will be heavier and more disruptive than they and their family can support. Or they may fear that surgery will leave them with unsightly scars. Or even that a clinic may be experimenting on blacks. ("Remember Tuskegee. I don't trust them.") I've even had patients express the fear that a neighbor or church member who works at the hospital might find out about his or her case and spread the word: "Child, she'll look at my chart."

I don't believe that doctors do much to vanquish these fears simply by repeating again and again that blacks are more likely both to get cancer and to die of it than whites, though this is true in a wide range of cancers. Such repeating does little good without action.

Some of the needed actions are obvious:

- Improving the socioeconomic status of blacks would help free our minds to focus on health matters.
- Including blacks in research projects both as researchers and as subjects would yield new discoveries about genetic and racial differences in the causes of cancer and responses to treatment.
- Providing full access to care that includes prompt diagnosis and therapy would have immediate benefits, and it must be sought and fought for.

WHAT YOU CAN DO FOR YOURSELF AND FOR OTHERS

Yes, there are health disparities over which you have little control. But the most important agent for lowering cancer incidence and mortality is the individual black man and black woman. The revolution in black health can begin here, today, with you. You joined this revolution when you picked up this book and began your education. And you extend this revolution when you assume responsibility for changing your own lifestyle, and spread the word to those around you. For the black woman and man in America, this is the all-important political act. Without our good health, after all, we can hardly be agents of other social change.

Responsibility for one's own health must be an essential goal—a moral and even a political goal.

There are injustices in the medical system that can prevent poor people, and sometimes simply black people, from getting the prompt and effective treatment that they need. That's why we all must continue the fight for access rights. Responsibility for one's own health must be an essential goal for our people—a moral and even a political goal.

At the same time, each of us can become part of this struggle simply by learning for ourselves and teaching others such health basics as:

- What symptoms to look for
- How often to have a general physical
- How often to have a manmogram, prostate, rectal or sidmoi-doscope exam
- The dangers of tobacco, smoked or chewed
- The fundamentals of good diet.

And each of us can take it upon himself or herself to help organize health fairs to spread the necessary knowledge.

Our first order of business, then, is to become responsible for our own health and the health of our children and loved ones, and to encourage others to do the same. More specifically:

- African Americans must quit smoking and discourage their children from acquiring a deadly habit. More than 20 percent of our people smoke. That one step alone would do much to reduce their chances of getting cancer of the lungs, esophagus, pancreas, kidney, and bladder. As matters stand, tobacco is responsible for about 20 percent of all cancer deaths. Many of us, that means, are simply committing suicide.
- African Americans must improve their diets. Planting a garden and eating the vegetables grandma fed us—carrots, beans, and collard greens—would improve our chance of not getting cancer. Trimming the fat off meat and eliminating the skin on chicken would put African Americans still further ahead.
- African Americans need physical activity and fitness and the weight reduction that follows from regular exercise. Exercise can help reduce the incidence of colon and breast cancer, and, of course, it greatly benefits the heart as well.

"How can you teach me?" the old gospel song asks. One answer, I think, is that we can spread the word about health in the African-American churches. We need to think of our bodies as "temples of the Holy Spirit," in His view, and we must maintain that temple by proper diet and exercise, and by avoiding substances like tobacco, alcohol, and hard drugs, substances that can bring the temple down as surely as Samson did.

Because maintaining our health, in Dr. Hamilton's view, is a religious responsibility, the church should promote and sponsor health fairs and seminars, and provide transportation to medical facilities. Other African-American organizations—Urban League, NAACP, and fraternities and sororities—should join forces with the church to educate black citizens. But ultimately each black citizen, each black family, must shed the cocoon of ignorance, fatalism, and suspicion, and take responsibility for his or her own health.

This book has three parts. In the first part, you will learn:

- Why cancer is of special importance to blacks
- Basic knowledge about cancer itself and what you can do to prevent it, and
- Areas of research that give us hope for the future.

The second part of the book describes the major cancers that affect African Americans, along with the symptoms and treatment of these diseases. Through that discussion, and by presenting typical personal cases, I want to shatter the mystery that surrounds those cancers so that we as a people can move on to enjoy the fruits of a healthy and dynamic life unencumbered by myth and ignorance.

The final part of the book takes up some of the many human questions that cancer patients have to wrestle with—questions such as:

- How do I get the best possible medical care and the best possible nonmedical support teams?
- How can body and mind work together to help me through treatment and recovery?

- How do I live with cancer on a day-to-day basis, and, if this should become necessary, how can I die with it in peace and dignity?

This book contains hard truths. But it also contains truths that bring comfort. The human spirit can be invincible—strong enough to allow people to hold their heads high even while they are fighting with cancer.

TWO

What Is Cancer?

BEFORE TELLING YOU WHAT CANCER IS, I want to say a word or two about why it's so serious a worry. For one thing, cancer can run in families. This means that certain people—about one in ten of all cases, no matter what their diet or exposure to other secondary causes of cancer—are born at risk. For another thing, cancer is a major disease that the latest data says is the second leading cause of death in the United States, taking more than half a million people according to the latest data.

The picture for African Americans is in some ways still bleaker. The most common cancers in men are cancers of the lung, colon and rectum, and prostate. These cancers, unfortunately, are more common in blacks, who also are more likely to die of them.

In women, breast cancer is the most common form, and it occurs in one person in nine. Although this particular form of cancer occurs less frequently in blacks, it tends to develop at an earlier age. And, again, the death rate among black woman with breast cancer is higher than among white women, in part because black women often get diagnosed later and are likely to have poorer access to health care than white women. Let's start changing this by learning what cancer is.

HOW CANCER WORKS

Cancer occurs because the cells run wild. For reasons we only partially understand, molecular defects in cells begin to send signals that result in unrestricted growth. These signals also attract additional blood vessels to the area, providing the "wild" cells with increased nutrients and oxygen that help them carry the cancer to other places in the body.

The new cancer cells, if they spread to a new, attractive home, multiply and grow. This process is repeated many times, and is repeated in many organs of the body. The invading cancer cells interfere with the functions of the organ they've made their new home. Like marauders, they cause devastation.

Eventually, as tissues expand from the cancerous growth and nerves become irritated by the sheer number and mass of invading cells, the patient feels pain. If the cancer cells develop in the lung, they may cause a cough, with or without blood. If they move into the kidney, bloody urine will result. In the liver, they create jaundice; in the brain, headache and, eventually, stupor. If the primary tumor is not removed before the spread begins, or if the secondary spread (metastases) is not controlled, death may result.

Cancer occurs because cells run wild.

The key question researchers have about cancer is what exactly sets the process going in the first place, and why does a particular person get cancer at a particular time. When we know this, we will be well on our way toward effective prevention and cure.

Today, we do know a good deal about the conditions and irritants (we call them *risk factors*) that *can* lead to cancer. Not all these risk factors are avoidable, but many of them are. Even if your genes make you vulnerable to cancer, there is still a great deal you can do to avoid ever getting it.

RISK FACTORS THAT CAN LEAD TO CANCER

While for some cancers we can't explain the cause, in some types people can be born with genetic defects that predispose them to cancer. People can also make life choices that make them potential cancer patients. Both types of conditions we call "risk factors." Several risk factors can lead to the development of cancer:

- Cancer can develop from a genetic defect. This defect may be very specific—a single gene in a single chromosome that gets passed on from generation to generation. Often, that misplaced gene blocks a protective

  Risk factors can lead to the development of cancer.

  mechanism in the cell. Cancer of the breast, ovary, colon, and some other cancers can result from a genetic defect.
- Obesity can cause cancer. Fat cells serve as reservoirs for calories the body can't use. New cells form and old cells expand to make room for excess fat. Once formed, these cells do not recede. (We sometimes call this process a *ratchet effect* because a ratchet turns always in one direction.) These reservoir cells may release some of their fat and return to normal size, but their number doesn't decrease, and it will increase if the fat intake increases. As it increases, so does the danger of cancer.
- Cigarette smoking causes 87 percent of lung cancer cases and is a major risk factor for many other cancers as well.
- Overexposure to the sun can cause skin cancer.
- Overexposure to radiation can cause cancer. (Many Japanese exposed to fallout from the atomic bomb developed leukemia and other cancers, and there is evidence that American nuclear workers similarly were exposed to abnormally high risk of these diseases.) Radiation of the head and neck in children may produce cancer of the thyroid later in life. Radiation appears to be dangerous in two ways: (1) it can act directly on

individual cells, making them cancerous, and (2) it may sup-press the body's defense system against tumor formation and at the same time promote the process that causes tissues to become cancerous.

- Overexposure to environmental toxins can cause cancer. Such toxins are in the air we breathe, the water we drink, and the soil we grow crops on. They are also sometimes in the foods we eat.

Cancer occurs because something causes the cells to change, but we don't know exactly how that change is triggered. In some types of cancer, we can identify particular irritants that set the process in motion. In lung cancer, it's easy: in 87 percent of the cases, tobacco is the culprit. In cancer of the cervix, herpes simplex type II and a virus called *papilloma* are the cause. In stomach cancer, smoked fish and the form of anemia we label "pernicious" stimulate the changes in the cell that lead to cancer. Soot seems to trigger cancer in the scrotum, which, not surprisingly, occurs mostly in chimney sweeps. Though we can identify irritants that stimulate cell changes, we don't know the mechanics of the triggering change itself.

WHAT PROTECTS THE BODY FROM CANCER

Just as we can identify substances and conditions that cause cancer, we know something about those that help prevent it by helping the body resist the changes in the cells that start the process. A person lessens his or her risk of skin cancer by avoiding long exposures to the sun. A smoker greatly improves his odds against getting lung cancer simply by stopping smoking. Those who continue to smoke despite their knowledge that it is "killing them softly," should know that smoking reduces levels of antioxidant nutrients. This means that smokers especially need to eat fruits and vegetables that con-tain those nutrients, and to take beta-carotene supplements in the

TABLE 2
Causes of Cancer by Type

TYPE OF CANCER	CAUSES OF CANCER
Lung, mouth, throat, esophagus	Tobacco
Breast	Obesity; high-fat diet; excessive estrogen
Cervix	HIV; Human papilloma virus (HPV)
Colon	The often unhealthy American diet; genetic mutation
Stomach	Smoked food; highly salted foods; the often unhealthy American diet; and HPI (H pylori infection)
Skin	Excess exposure to the sun
Skin, esophagus, stomach, cervix	HIV
Skin, lymphoma	HIV; excessive exposure to the sun
Liver	Hepatitis B and C
Lung, bladder, lining of chest cavity	Asbestosis
Thyroid, leukemia	Radiation
Breast, colon, ovary	Genetic mutation
Mouth, esophagus	Alcohol; tobacco
Leukemia, sarcoma, lymphoma	Viruses

form of pills, and vitamins C and E. In fact, diets high in fresh fruits and vegetables are good for all of us. Building up our antioxidant nutrients is one way to keep cancer away from our door.

If certain genes make it more likely that a particular person will get cancer, there are other genes—we call them *suppressor genes*—that make it *less* likely. A gene that has been labeled the p53 gene, for example, protects the body against cancer of the lung, breast, colon, and bone. How it does this is too complicated to explain here, but I can say simply that it works through a complex mechanism of checks and balances that control the way the body's cells and organs work with one another.

Playing Safe by Screening

The American Cancer Society (ACS) recommends the following guidelines for people at average risk for cancer who have no specific symptoms. People at increased risk for certain cancers may need to be screened at an earlier age or to be screened more often. Should you or a loved one show symptoms that could be related to cancer, see a doctor right away.

A checkup for cancer should be part of your regular health examination. (If you don't have a doctor, talk to a social worker or health care provider about how you can get that regular examination.) A cancer-related checkup should include health counseling and, depending on your age, might include examinations for breast cancer and cancers of the thyroid, oral cavity, skin, lymph nodes, testes, and ovaries, as well as for some non-malignant diseases.

The ACS recommends tests for specific cancer sites as outlined below.

BREAST CANCER

- Yearly mammograms should start at age forty and continue for as long as a woman is in good health.

- Clinical breast exams (CBE) should be part of a periodic health exam, about every three years for women in their twenties and thirties, and every year for women forty and over.
- Women should report any breast change promptly to their health care providers. Breast self-exam (BSE) is an option for women, starting in their twenties.
- Women at increased risk (e.g., because of family history, genetic tendency, or past breast cancer) should talk with their doctors about the benefits and limitations of starting mammography screening earlier, having additional tests (e.g., breast ultrasound or MRI), or having more frequent exams.

COLON AND RECTAL CANCER

Beginning at age fifty, both men and women at average risk for developing colorectal cancer should follow one of these five testing schedules:

- Yearly fecal occult blood test (FOBT)* or fecal immunochemical test (FIT)
- Flexible sigmoidoscopy every five years
- Yearly FOBT* or FIT plus flexible sigmoidoscopy every five years**
- Double-contrast barium enema every five years
- Colonoscopy every ten years.

All positive tests should be followed up with colonoscopy.

People should begin colorectal cancer screening earlier and/or undergo screening more often if they have any of the following colorectal cancer risk factors.

- A personal history of colorectal cancer or adenomatous polyps (a type of colon polyp)
- A strong family history of colorectal cancer or polyps (cancer or polyps in a first-degree relative younger than sixty or in two first-degree relatives of any age) Note: a first degree relative is defined as a parent, sibling, or child.

---

* For FOBT, the take-home multiple sample method should be used.

** The combination of yearly FOBT or FIT plus flexible sigmoidoscopy every five years is preferred over either of these options alone.

- A personal history of chronic inflammatory bowel disease
- A family history of an hereditary colorectal cancer syndrome (familial adenomatous polyposis or hereditary nonpolyposis colon cancer).

CERVICAL CANCER
The American Cancer Society also recommends:

- All women should begin cervical cancer screening about three years after they begin having vaginal intercourse, but no later than when they are twenty-one years old. Screening should be done every year with the regular Pap test or every two years using the newer liquid-based Pap test.
- Beginning at age thirty, women who have had three normal Pap test results in a row may get screened every two to three years with either the conventional (regular) or liquid-based Pap test. Women who have certain risk factors such as diethyl-stilbestrol (DES) exposure before birth, HIV infection, or a weakened immune system due to organ transplant, chemotherapy, or chronic steroid use should continue to be screened annually.
- Another reasonable option for women over thirty is to get screened every three years (but not more frequently) with either the conventional or liquid-based Pap test, *plus* the HPV DNA test.
- Women seventy years of age or older who have had three or more normal Pap tests in a row and no abnormal Pap test results in the last ten years may choose to stop having cervical cancer screening. Women with a history of cervical cancer, DES exposure before birth, HIV infection, or a weakened immune system should continue to have screening as long as they are in good health.

Women who have had a total hysterectomy (removal of the uterus and cervix) may also choose to stop having cervical cancer screening, unless the surgery was done as a treatment for cervical cancer or precancer. Women who have had a hysterectomy without removal of the cervix should continue to follow the guidelines above.

ENDOMETRIAL (UTERINE) CANCER
The American Cancer Society recommends that all women should
be informed about the risks and symptoms of endometrial cancer, and strongly encouraged to report any unexpected bleeding
or spotting to their doctors. For women with or at high risk for
hereditary nonpolyposis colon cancer (HNPCC), annual screening
should be offered for endometrial cancer with endometrial
biopsy beginning at age thirty-five.

PROSTATE CANCER
Both the prostate-specific antigen (PSA) blood test and digital
rectal examination (DRE) should be offered annually, beginning
at age fifty, to men who have at least a ten-year life expectancy.
Men at high risk (African-American men and men with a strong
family history of one or more first-degree relatives—father,
brothers—diagnosed at an early age) should begin testing at
age forty-five. Men at even higher risk, due to multiple first-
degree relatives affected at an early age, could begin testing at
age forty. Depending on the results of this initial test, no further
testing might be needed until age forty-five.

  Information should be provided to all men about what is
known and what is uncertain about the benefits and limitations
of early detection and treatment of prostate cancer so that they
can make an informed decision about testing.

  Men who ask their doctor to make the decision on their
behalf should be tested. Discouraging testing is not appropriate.
Also, not offering testing is not appropriate.

REFERENCE
American Cancer Society. *Cancer Facts & Figures 2005*. Atlanta,
GA: American Cancer Society, 2005.

SOME QUESTIONS AND SOME ANSWERS

Suppressor genes make cancer less likely.

Let's end this chapter with a question-and-answer session. The questioner is one of my patients. I'll call her Mary Hall. Her mother died of cancer, and so did two of her aunts. She's lived in fear of the disease for a long time, fear that kept her from seeing me. But now, finally, with a little prodding from her son and daughter, she's come in for an examination.

Mary is a little embarrassed. She doesn't have any symptoms and isn't convinced she needs to talk to a doctor. I've been busy telling her that she shouldn't feel embarrassed—just the opposite. The fact is, she's practicing preventive medicine, which is, in my mind, the best medicine there is. And now she's ready to ask me some excellent questions.

Q. With somebody like me, who doesn't have the disease—at least, I hope I don't. . . . I know you want to do some tests. What's the first symptom I have to look for?

A. First, I want to say that you've come in at just the right time. Most likely we'll find nothing wrong. But sometimes in an examination we can catch cancers in their early stage, when they're most treatable. These are often cancers you won't discover yourself because, if the cancer is in a very early stage, you won't feel any symptoms.

Q. How can that be? I mean, if I've got a tumor in me, surely I would feel some symptoms.

A. Well, the fact is that tumors can be very small—too small to see with the eye or feel with the hand. If we do catch them early, by means of x-ray images, for example, they're easy to remove, and often that means there won't be further trouble.

That's why we do tests—to catch these things before you do, to catch what you might miss during your self-examinations, for many cancer symptoms don't show up early. When they finally do show up, the disease is at a more advanced stage. At that point, treatment becomes more complicated and more chancy. The earlier symptoms are diagnosed, the better.

Q. Tell me, then, how do you go about finding things in my body that I haven't found myself?

A. That depends. For breast cancer, what we see is a small shadow on an x-ray picture or on some other image of the interior of your breast. When that shadow turns out to represent a tumor that can't be palpated—that is, felt—we may have an early sign of breast cancer.

Q. What about other kinds of cancers? Do you have tests for them?

A. Yes, we do. For example, we can identify cervical cancer, or the changes that lead to it, by doing a Pap smear. That's another test women need to have done regularly each year. For a number of cancers, we can actually see inside you with a flexible light. In some cases, with a cutting instrument attached to that light, we can remove small clusters of precancerous or cancerous cells without needing to perform surgery.

But an informed patient can watch for warning signs. This does not mean living in fear. It just means keeping an eye on certain symptoms or changes in the body that might occur.

The American Cancer Society notes six warning signs of cancer. Here they are:

• A sore that doesn't heal
• Unusual bleeding or discharge
• Thickening or a lump in the breast or other part of the body
• Indigestion or difficulty in swallowing
• Obvious change in wart or mole
• Nagging cough or hoarseness.

Q. I guess I know part of the answer to this one already, but I'll
    ask. What's the picture at the next stage, if you don't detect the
    cancer early?

A. Even when cancer isn't caught in its earliest stage, treatment is
    still possible, and often it's successful. But I need to repeat:
    we'd much rather catch the cancer early—nip the thing in the
    bud.

Q. O.K. It hurts me to think that if my ma and my aunts had
    understood that, they'd be here today. But I understand it, and
    my daughter will understand it, too. So I guess that's progress.

A. It sure is. It means that in one family, at least, we can change
    the pattern and save lives.

Q. I'm going to ask you another question. I heard that if air gets
    to a tumor, it can spread.

A. No, Mary, that's a common belief, but it's not true. People
    sometimes believe this because they find out after a biopsy that
    the cancer has spread. But neither the biopsy nor the air causes
    that.

Q. Well, that's a relief. I remember my aunt told me that's why she
    never did go in for a biopsy. But I have another question that
    worries me: when does a tumor become incurable?

A. Yes, that's a tough one. The general answer is when vital struc-
    tures like the heart and brain get invaded. Severe pain or even
    paralysis is a pretty sure sign the cancer is incurable. Pain or
    paralysis means that major nerves have been affected.

Where that pain occurs depends on the location of the cancer. If
the cancer is in the cervix and rectum, the nerves in the lower back
may be involved. If it's in the pancreas, the nerves in the middle of the
back may register pain. Lung cancer, if it isn't caught in time, may
invade the nerves of the chest, arm, or neck. And breast cancer can
spread so as to attach to the chest walls and then to the ribs.

These late stage tumors can have other symptoms as well. The
tumor may become ulcerated and infected, and cause fever or anemia

and weakness. Anemia (low blood count) is common when cancer hits the part of the colon near the appendix—the part we call the *cecum.* Sometimes this is mistaken for appendicitis or gallbladder disease. We can cure or control the infection in these cases, but the tumor still needs to be treated and removed.

A cancer can cause symptoms that make diagnosis difficult.

A cancer can also cause symptoms that make diagnosis difficult. The tumor itself can produce hormones or other substances. For example, a lung cancer can produce cortisone, which is ordinarily produced only in the adrenal gland. A tumor of the testicle may produce thyroid hormone. These abnormal secretions sometimes present us doctors with a bizarre and puzzling clinical picture.

Q. So my kids were right making me come in today? If I'm going to have to get treatment, I'd certainly prefer to get it at that early stage before things get so complicated.

A. Yes, that's the important lesson. You know, even at the later stages, we can lessen suffering and save lives. But what you've learned is what I pray everyone might learn: *the key is to detect the tumor early and initiate early and effective treatment.* What this means for you, Mary, is that you need to be aware of your body and alert to changes.

Even more important, you need to stay healthy—that means watching what you eat, controlling your weight by exercising, examining your own breasts once a month, and coming in to see me for a complete physical exam once a year.

DISPELLING CANCER MYTHS

Here is a list of common beliefs about cancer *that aren't true.* I include them because I've known patients who believed them, and because they believed them, they sought help and were diagnosed and treated too late.

- If air gets to cancer, as in a biopsy or operation, the cancer will spread as a result.
- Cancer is "folly of the devil"—that is, caused by the devil.
- Some cancers are "eating cancers"—that is, in spreading they eat tissue away.
- Blacks don't get skin cancer (melanoma). (It's rare in blacks, but it does occur.)
- Clinical trials are just experimentation.
- Cancer is a death sentence.
- Mastectomy takes away a woman's femininity and makes her less sexy.
- Discharge from the nipples always means cancer.
- A rash around a nipple doesn't mean cancer unless there is also a tumor.
- Having a hysterectomy before menopause can decrease a woman's sexual desires.

THREE

Diet and Prevention

ATING A GOOD DIET helps determine your state of health, the range of activities you engage in, how a child grows, and how you respond to the illnesses and stresses of everyday life. Some health choices by you or a parent can follow you all your life—for example, whether your first meal is breast milk or formula. Feeding breast milk means better nourishment, better resistance to disease, and may even help develop higher intelligence and greater emotional stability.

Of course, what we eat and how we eat is in part determined by our cultural backgrounds and also by our economic status. But in the end the choice is ours. We don't have to eat in the same way our parents did. You can find useful diet tips along with delicious and healthy soul food recipes at *www.hiltonpub.com* and in *The Heart of the Matter* by Hilton M. Hudson II, M.D., F.A.C.S., and Herbert Stern, Ph.D. (Hilton Publishing Company, Chicago, IL.) and at the American Dietician Association Web site (*www.eatright.org*). Eat right, get regular exercise, and don't smoke—there's a formula for not getting cancer.

The obesity epidemic in the United States is not about body "styles" that black men or black women may or may not like. It is about increased heart disease, hypertension, stroke, diabetes and arthritis. Some studies find that certain cancers—endometrial, esophagus, colon, breast, and kidney are also more likely to occur in overweight people.

Every five years the United States Department of Health and Human Services in conjunction with the U.S. Department of Agriculture publishes *Dietary Guidelines for Americans*. The last set of recommendations was published in 2005 and used the pyramid as its new logo to emphasize the various food groups making up a healthy diet and the proper proportions for each group. Also notice the healthy-looking figure climbing the pyramid.

The core recommendations of the guidelines are as follows:

- Eat a variety of foods.

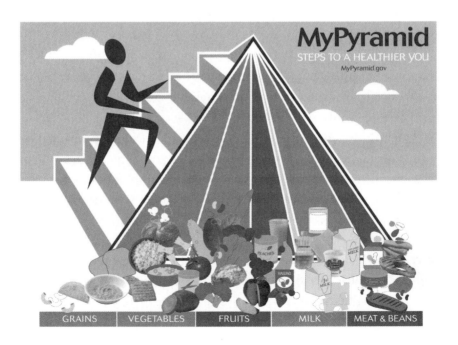

- Maintain a healthy body weight. A general rule of thumb is to maintain your weight within 5 pounds of your weight when you were twenty years old.
- Engage in regular physical activity.

For more details, you can download the National Institute of Health's pamphlet, *Dietary Guidelines for Americans,* at *www. healthierus.gov/dietaryguidelines/.* The pamphlet is free. The upshot is that you can avoid many serious diseases just by taking good care of yourself.

Because the relationship between diet and cancer is complex, we seem to be bombarded with new recommendations almost weekly. One week scientific literature reports that a high-fat diet leads to breast cancer; the next week another report finds that a high-fat diet makes little difference in the cancer rate. So on that score, though we don't have final answers, you are best off to bet on the safe side. Adherence to guidelines indisputably reduces the risk of chronic disease, particularly cardiovascular disease.

Today, much of the scientific community holds that a diet that includes vegetables, fruits, and whole grains reduces the risk for colorectal, oral, and esophageal cancers. Red meats and diets high in animal fats are associated with an increase in cancers of the colon and prostate. A high-fat diet has also been linked to breast cancer.

Each person, with the help of a health care professional or dietician, if possible, has to work out his or her own proper diet. The choice will take in factors like height, weight, age at first menstruation, growth rate, and a variety of other data. The trick is to find the point where most of the energy you consume is being burned off in activity, and as little as possible stored as body fat. Dietary fat has the highest energy content of all the nutrients, at nine calories per gram. Carbohydrate and protein provide 4 calories per gram. Reducing dietary fat reduces body weight.

A high-fiber diet has historically been associated with a lower incidence of colon cancer. High-fiber diets are the norm in developing countries, where the incidence of colon cancers is low measured against the rates in industrialized countries. Today, newer studies are casting a shadow over whether a diet high in fiber provides protection. Current scientific thought looks not so much at single factors as to single factors in the context of other factors, including activity level, energy balance, and the protective effects of fresh fruit and vegetables.

While health is obviously a personal or family concern, we must also suggest that it is a racial concern. Disparity in African-American health begins with the diet and nutritional status of mothers. The percent of low birth weight infants in African Americans is 13.29 percent versus 6.8 percent in whites (2002). Too often, these low birth weight infants grow to be "thick" adults. Fifty percent of African-American women are overweight, and disparity in diet often exists for a lifetime. Changing eating habits must occur over a sustained period of time in order to make significant change. Quick diet fixes don't work in the long-run.

We all know that poor communities don't have access to well-stocked grocery stores, though we can find plenty of corner convenience stores that sell cigarettes, candy, lottery tickets, and other various sundries, along with unhealthy fast foods or a few sorry vegetables and meat you can't be too sure about. That's a good reason to drive, get on a bus, or even take a cab with neighbors and get to the nearest big grocery store once a week or so. In that way you're more likely to eat foods that are healthy and fresh.

Southern cooking style predominates in the African-American home. Fried foods, cooked greens, and high-fat-content meats, such as sausage, bacon, ribs, are traditional. Adopting a healthier diet is possible, but requires culturally competent approaches. Again, the recipes at *www.hiltonpub.com* will show you how to satisfy yourself and your family with meals that aren't dangerous to your health.

We recommend that you read food labels on canned and packaged food you buy. Making yourself aware of what you are putting into your stomach is a good start for changing your diet. And keep

Your Guide: Read the Food Label

Food labels can help you choose foods lower in sodium, as well as calories, saturated fat, total fat, and cholesterol. The label tells you:

NUMBER OF SERVINGS
The serving size is $\frac{1}{2}$ cup. The package contains about 3 servings.

AMOUNT PER SERVING
Nutrient amounts are given for one serving. If you eat more or less than a serving, add or subtract amounts. For example, if you eat 1 cup of peas, you need to double the nutrient amounts on the label.

PERCENT DAILY VALUE
Percent Daily Value helps you compare products and tells you if the food is high or low in sodium. Choose products with the lowest Percent Daily Value for sodium.

Frozen Peas

Serving Size: 1/2 cup (68 g)
Servings Per Container: about 3

Amount Per Serving

Calories 60	Calories from Fat 0
	% Daily Value*
Total Fat 0 g	0%
Saturated Fat 0 g	0%
Cholesterol 0 mg	0%
Sodium 125 mg	5%
Total Carbohydrate 11 g	4%
Dietary Fiber 6 g	22%
Sugars 5 g	
Protein 5 g	
Vitamin A 15%	Vitamin C 30%
Calcium 0%	Iron 6%

* Percent Daily Values are based on a 2,000 calorie diet.

NUTRIENTS
You'll find the milligrams of sodium in one serving.

Source: National Heart, Lung, and Blood Institute, rover.nhlbi.nih.gov/cgi-bin/search?site=NHLBI_Public&client=NHLBI_Public_frontend&proxystylesheet=NHLBI_Public_frontend&output=xml_no_dtd&getfields=description.keywords&q=food+label+%2B+how+to+read&btnG.x=0&btnG.y=0&btnG=Go

in mind that some African-American standards, such as collard and mustard greens, corn bread, grits, and yams are good for you.

EXERCISE

Again, diet alone can't prevent cancer. It has to be thought of together with regular, adequate exercise. Think of what we eat as fuel, and what we burn off as energy. If we put in more food than we burn off in exercise, we gain weight. One of the first factors ever identified with cancer prevention was weight control. Thin animals lived longer and developed tumors less often then heavy animals. While research goes on, we believe that the same is true of human beings.

We all know, or maybe even have said, the common excuses for *not* exercising: "I get enough exercise at work," "I just don't have the time," "My body is too weak for me to get started." Remember that the exercise you do at work isn't always the kind that's good for your body, that very busy people *make* time because they know that the quality of their lives, and maybe life itself, depends on it. As for weakness, it doesn't matter where you are when you start exercising. If you're too weak to walk to the corner, at least walk down and up your stairs. Even mild exercise, if you do it regularly, will make you ready for more strenuous exercise.

People find lots of different ways to exercise. Some like to go to a gym and be guided by a trainer. Some like sports, or energy-burning exercises like jogging, or swimming, or playing sports. And others simply walk, starting with what they can do without straining, and gradually working up. That's something you can do alone, or with a spouse or neighbor. And if your neighborhood doesn't feel safe for walking, try a mall, or a safe nearby park. Your goal is to walk two miles in thirty minutes on most days of the week. That is what is considered to be moderate activity. If you're trying to lose weight, take a walk three or more times a week or as prescribed by a health care professional. Chronic diseases like arthritis, diabetes, or a heart condition will limit the exercise you can do. But everyone, the strong and the weak, the healthy and the ill, can find an exercise that suits their condition, even if that exercise means no more than sitting up in bed or walking to the bathroom.

Minerals, such as calcium, selenium, vitamins C, A, E, and more recently folate, and pharmaceutical approaches, including aspirin and other anti-inflammatory medications, continue to be studied in large clinical trials. But, to date, the results haven't been encouraging. A pill that can prevent cancer is something all of us, including the pharmaceutical companies, are looking for. However, for the time being at least, it doesn't exist—and even if it did, there's no substitute for a healthy diet, adequate exercise, and not smoking or living unhealthy lifestyles.

FOUR

Current Research: Paths into the Future

W E HAVE ALREADY TALKED about two aspects of cancer that allow for optimism. The first is early diagnosis, which gives you an excellent chance of recovery and cure. The second is prevention. True, not all cancers are preventable, but we can avoid life choices that make us more vulnerable to cancer.

In this chapter, we turn to a third source of optimism. Cancer has the attention of some of the best minds in medical research. In the coming decades, our knowledge about cancer in general, and breast cancer in particular, will grow rapidly. New knowledge will mean new treatments that are physically and emotionally easier on patients and more likely to ensure cure than anything we have today.

THE CAUSES OF CANCER

The war against cancer takes place on two main fronts. The first is the daily choices the patient makes to strengthen or weaken the body. The second is the continuing scientific exploration into the genetic, chemical, and molecular processes that set cancer in motion, along with the pursuit of more accurate ways of detecting cancer and more efficient ways of treating it.

Some of that research will certainly pay off in the coming years, and we watch the studies with great interest.

CLINICAL TRIALS

In a clinical trial, certain patients choose to be treated with a new drug or procedure. Obviously, new drugs and procedures developed in laboratories must be tested outside those laboratories. Although testing on animals can be helpful in the early stages, ultimately tests must be done on humans to find out if the treatment is effective.

In the case of breast cancer, African-American women must be included in the sample population. That is the only way that experimenters can determine whether the causes, and therefore the treatment, of cancer may in specific ways be different for African-American women than for Caucasian women.

Though what I've been saying sounds innocent enough, you, as an African-American reader, will see at once that something remains unsaid. We all know that in the past, in such experiments as the notorious one that took place at Tuskegee, black people were used in medical experimentation without regard to their health or even their lives. The aftershock of those experiments is still with us. Black people are reluctant to participate in experimental medical programs lest they again become victims to them.

Speaking as an African-American doctor, I can only say that Tuskegee is behind us. Certainly, treatment with new drugs and new medical procedures involves risks. But for patients who have exhausted the more conventional treatments, experimental methods may

Tuskegee is behind us.

offer a chance where there was none. Further, *by becoming part of clinical trials, patients get the opportunity to be part of the fight against cancer.* The very clinical trial you participate in could result in some breakthrough therapy, or lessen the side effects of a therapy already in use.

African-American patients will be most comfortable participating where there are African-American investigators involved in all aspects of the trial. But even where this is not the case, patients are often able to feel secure. The sad fact is that at present there is a shortage of African-American women represented in these test populations, and, in some cases, this means that African-American women are denied the most promising treatments. In a clinical trial, some patients are treated in the established ways, whereas others are given the new treatment. That way, the benefit of a new drug or procedure can be weighed against the benefit of the old ones.

Not all patients who volunteer for such trials are eligible. Each trial will be aimed at patients with very specific medical conditions. One trial may be open only to cases where cancer hasn't spread to the lymph nodes. Another, to cases in which cancer hasn't spread to body organs like the liver or brain.

Only the patient herself or her loved ones, with the counsel of her physician, can decide whether a particular trial is suitable for her. It is always the patient's option to opt out for any reason. That may mean that she is not satisfied with the results, or that she is bothered by the side effects, or even that she simply no longer wishes to be part of an experiment. The more the patient understands about the specific procedure and the desired outcome, the more comfortable she is likely to be with the experimental nature of these clinical trials.

YOUR RIGHT TO KNOW

Until quite recently, doctors would decide what was best for their patients, and patients would simply follow their doctor's advice. Although this may continue to be the path followed by many of us, there are also many patients today who, by reading and searching the Internet, research their own treatment options.

On the whole, *we think that the more a patient knows about the options, the better his or her treatment is likely to go.* At the same time, the patient's research should be carried out in a cooperative spirit with the physician. The doctor's own recommendations should be the crucial factor in the patient's decision, although he or she may, and probably should, seek a second opinion, a subject I'll say more about later in this book.

> *The patient's research should be carried out in a cooperative spirit with the physician.*

Your choice of treatment may sometimes be determined simply by your temperament. Some treatments mean longer periods of uncertainty than others. Some may involve calculated risks. Only you can decide your own tolerance for uncertainty and risk.

If you decide to do research on your own, a good place to start is the National Cancer Institute's Web site at *www.cancer.gov*. You can learn more about clinical trials at *www.cancer.gov/clinicaltrials.*

PART II

Types of Cancer, Symptoms, Diagnosis, Treatment

FIVE

Breast Cancer

TUESDAY NIGHT, after she put the kids to bed, Rebecca enjoyed her shower. Then, before she got into her nightgown, she examined her breasts, as she'd gotten used to doing once a month. But this time, to her dismay, she felt a "knot" in her right breast. It was small enough, but she knew it didn't belong there.

Worried, she called me that night, and after calming her as well as I could, I told her to come to my office the next morning, just before my regular office hours. There, in my examination room, I found what she had found: a mass the size of a walnut in her right breast.

Not all lumps in the breast are cancerous. Some are simply cysts. But cysts are pliable, and her lump didn't have the consistency of a cyst. The only way I could be sure, however, was to try to remove fluid from the mass (we call this *aspiration*). If it turned out to be a cyst, it would be full of liquid.

Unfortunately, as far as I could tell at this stage, it appeared not to be. Rebecca agreed to a second step: this time I took a tiny sample of the mass through a simple procedure called *needle aspiration biopsy*, and sent it to the pathology lab, where they could study the cells. Rebecca would have to wait a few days for their findings. I knew what that was like, having gone through such a wait myself, and I comforted and encouraged her as best I could.

Not all lumps in the breast are cancerous.

The news I gave her when she returned that Friday wasn't good. The pathology report read "suspicious for cancer." This meant that individual cells in the needle aspiration biopsy sample appeared to be cancer cells, though we couldn't be positive until we'd examined an actual piece of the tumor. There were several other tests we needed to try. Some of them could show that our working hypothesis was wrong. That's how medical science works, patiently disentangling the net of possibilities in order to arrive at the one that seems most in keeping with the presented facts.

What we needed to do first, I told Rebecca, was to get a mammogram. She asked me why since we knew already that there was a tumor. The purpose of the mammogram, I told her, wasn't to diagnose the lump we'd already found. Instead, we wanted to see if there were other areas in either breast that we needed to look at. If other areas were found, they would have to be removed and examined using a procedure called a *biopsy*.

When I'd examined Rebecca, I hadn't felt any tumors in her lymph nodes. The lymph nodes are bean-shaped organs that serve as kinds of centers for the lymphatic vessels, as parts of a system essential to our ability to resist disease. These lymph nodes store cells that trap and fight cancer cells and bacteria. They're to be found in the underarms, chest, neck, groin, abdomen, and elsewhere. But I'd felt no tumors there. The mammogram, too, was reassuring. As far as I could tell at this stage, Rebecca had only the one tumor she'd originally discovered.

"Rebecca," I said, "nobody wants to have cancer. If it were on the menu, it's not what you'd order. It is frightening to know that you have it, and it's frightening to think about going through long and mysterious treatments that may or may not work.

"But in your case, there's a lot to encourage us. It's possible that our diagnosis is wrong, though that's an outside chance. The more likely case is the cancer is local: it's only in the one spot you discovered. That means that we have some options in treating it. I'm going to lay them out for you, and I know you'll have questions to ask. You have some time, but the sooner we start treatment, the better. Once you have been treated, your chances of kicking this thing altogether—that is, of getting cured—are 80 percent or better."

Lymph nodes store cells that trap and fight cancer cells and bacteria.

OPTIONS FOR TREATMENT

Rebecca listened. These were the options I laid out to her:

1. The tumor could be cut out, along with a 1-inch "cuff" of normal tissue. We would remove that cuff because if the cancer turned out to be what we call a *frank* or *invasive cancer*, the cancerous cells would have invaded the floor of the tissue on which they rest. By examining the removed tumor and tissue, we could determine with fair accuracy whether the cancerous mass had been completely removed.

   At the same time that I removed the tumor and cuff, I would take a sample from her armpit (axilla) to see if the cancer had spread. This procedure is called *sentinel lymph-node sampling*.

   As a kind of insurance policy, after the patient has healed from surgery, x-ray treatment will follow, with or without chemical therapy (chemotherapy). Whether we use chemotherapy depends on what we find when we examine the removed specimen.

   If Rebecca chose this procedure, we'd arrange for her to talk to the radiation and chemotherapy doctors, who'd tell her

about the details of their treatments, the risks, and the side
effects. Rebecca was a patient who, step by step, wanted to
know what we were doing and why. (Maybe it's merely my
doctor's prejudice, but I find that patients who take that kind
of active interest in their disease do better in treatment.
Because they tend to be less frightened and less suspicious,
they can put more energy into surviving and getting well.)

2. Our second option would be to remove the entire breast. We
   call this a *modified radical mastectomy*. This means we'd
   remove the breast along with tissue in the armpit. Whether this
   procedure would be followed by chemotherapy would depend
   on whether the tumor had spread to the armpit or in other
   ways looked "aggressive."

3. The third option would be for Rebecca to enter a clinical trial.
   Some African-American patients refuse to enter these because
   of the bad history of experiments like those at Tuskegee many
   years ago. But in clinical trials like those I'm talking about, the
   patient is assured of getting a treatment that medical science
   thinks beneficial. These trials aim at finding out which treatments are *best* for which patients at various stages of cancer.
   The only way we can know this is by trying them and statistically analyzing the results.

In agreeing to be part of a test, as I encouraged her to, Rebecca
agreed that she'd enter a treatment program without knowing in
advance exactly what the treatment would be. It could involve
lumpectomy (the removal of the immediately diseased area) or
mastectomy (the removal of the entire breast). It could include x-ray
treatment with chemotherapy or x-ray treatment without it.

Rebecca chose to enter a clinical trial. Because clinical trials are
designed to weigh one recommended treatment against another one,
I was convinced, and I convinced her, that this would guarantee her
a strongly recommended treatment. I also knew that Rebecca had the
strength of mind to bear the uncertainty of not knowing which treat-

ment she was receiving. For the purpose of the test, that information is withheld both from the patient and from her physician.

Rebecca's decision rested in part on her wanting her treatment to contribute to knowledge that might save future cancer patients. She told me she was glad to feel she wasn't fighting just her cancer but everyone's. That thought helped her keep her spirits up during the whole ordeal. She understood that it might take years before the data from the study she'd been part of could be fully analyzed, but as she said to me, "That's O.K. I can wait that long."

I'm happy to say that Rebecca is doing well after two years. To be sure, we don't speak of a cure until a patient has been free of cancer for five years. But in my experience, the odds in Rebecca's favor are very good. Since her surgery and follow-up treatment, Rebecca has become a kind of cancer counselor in her church. She talks to her friends and anyone else who will listen about what they can do to avoid cancer, and about what doctors are doing in their fight to treat and cure it.

DIAGNOSIS

In talking about Rebecca's case, I've already told you something about diagnosis, but because it's a crucial subject, I want to tell you a bit more. You know already that early diagnosis is the best way to improve the chances of surviving breast cancer. It's also the best way to combat the soaring death rate as a result of breast cancer among African-American women. Until we have an actual cure, prevention and early detection must remain our main concern.

Cure will come one day in the form of gene therapy, or a pill that improves your immune system, or even an immunizing shot that prevents the disease. Till then, the "three-point play" set forth by the American Cancer Society and reported in the October 1999 issue of *Ebony* remains the most effective means of detecting breast cancer. It is supported not only by several groups of breast cancer survivors, but also by the Women's National Basketball Association (WNBA) and the National Medical Association (NMA), which is the African-American equivalent of the American Medical Association (AMA).

THE THREE-POINT PLAY

The three-point play is this simple:

1. Monthly self-exams of the breast
2. Breast exams by a physician once a year for women over forty years old
3. Annual mammograms.

Self-Examination

Self-examination, or palpation, though it's not entirely reliable, is the first necessary part of the diagnostic process. It's first because in my practice many cancers of the breast were first detected by the patient.

The American Cancer Society recommends that women practice breast self-examination monthly from the age of twenty. Start by choosing a specific date: the first of the month, or the day your menses begins. (If you tie the self-examination in with the beginning of your menstruation period, be sure to continue to practice it if you get pregnant. Yes, unfortunately, cancer *can* occur in the pregnant breast, and in fact, it grows rapidly because of the high level of hormones during pregnancy.)

In my practice, many cancers of the breast were first detected by the patient.

A good time to examine the breast is while you are taking a shower or bath. The soapy fingers are sensitive, and you are more likely under those conditions to detect a lump if a tumor is present. After a few such examinations, you will become familiar with the texture of your breast and know it better than anyone.

Palpating your breast is simple. Raise your arm on the side of the breast to be examined and place that hand behind your head. With the opposite hand, feel the armpit with a kneading motion to detect any lumps or lymph nodes. Remember, breast cancer may spread to the lymph glands in the armpit first, and you will want to discover this if it has occurred. It can be the earliest warning of all.

As to lumps, these *can* be produced by conditions that aren't in themselves cancerous. Some women develop a condition called *fibrocystic disease*, which though painful, is not dangerous. Common among teenagers, especially among African-American teenagers, is something

Examine the breast while you are taking a shower or bath.

called *fibroadenoma*. It is a firm, rubbery growth that your doctor will want to keep an eye on, but it usually doesn't require treatment unless it grows rapidly or becomes painful.

If a patient develops several fibroadenomas, my practice is to wait to remove them all at once when the patient turns twenty years old. Such growths *can* become cancerous, but this is rare.

We've been talking about what you can discover in the area of the breast and armpit. When you've finished examining the armpit, look at the nipple and the skin around it. Is there a rash? A cancer of the breast called *Paget's disease of the nipple* is first detected by a rash. This crusted and scaly rash causes the area of the nipple to redden, and sometimes to burn and itch. If it does not go away in a week after treatment with a bland salve, see your physician.

Now squeeze your nipples to see if there is a discharge. If there is, reexamine your nipple after a few days. If again there is a discharge, see your physician. If the discharge is bloody, see your physician the first time it occurs.

Though it's important that you see your doctor if you experience such discharges, most discharges, even if bloody, are *not* caused by cancer. A cyst may be spilling into a duct, or a small, benign, non-palpable tumor called an *adenoma* may be present in one of the ducts. But sometimes a malignancy is present, so it's essential that you get a medical evaluation.

Now that you've examined your nipples, palpate (that is, feel) your breast in a circular movement out from the nipple to the armpit in widening circles. If you notice an abnormality, repeat the exam weekly. If the abnormality persists for three weeks, see your doctor. Repeat this exam on the other breast.

One last suggestion. It is useful to keep a notebook in which you record the findings of these self-examinations. Your breast notebook will provide a clear record of the normal state of your breasts, so that should an abnormality appear, you will be tuned in to it at once.

The Clinical Breast Examination

A woman needs to get a breast exam every three years from the age of twenty to forty, and every year after that. If there is a strong family history of breast cancer, it's best to get an exam each year from the twenty-fifth year on. Many women schedule the breast exam for the same time as their annual Pap smears, and I recommend that plan.

The doctor's examination will be similar to your self-examination, though obviously it will feel different. Assuming that you have a relationship of trust with your physician, whether the doctor is male or female, you probably won't experience much self-consciousness. The doctor will repeat the steps you do at home. In addition, he or she will compare the breasts, noticing any differences in contour or in the retraction of the nipples. An underlying cancer may cause the skin to pucker or appear dimpled or the breast to appear flattened. A cancer may distort the shape of the nipple.

The doctor will also ask you to lean forward and compress your hands onto your hips. Again, this will help him or her to note any distortion in the breast.

The Mammogram

The mammogram is simply an x-ray of the breast. In a procedure common in this country since the early 1960s, a technician places your breasts between two plates and snaps an x-ray picture. It can often detect a mass too small to be felt—that is, as small as 1 cen-

FIGURE 2
MASSES IN THE BREAST

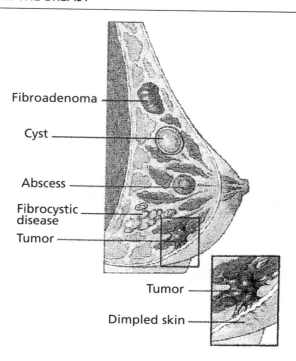

Fibroadenoma

Cyst

Abscess

Fibrocystic disease

Tumor

Tumor

Dimpled skin

timeter, or nearly 1/3 inch, which is how big it has to be before you or your doctor can detect it.

All women should have annual mammograms beginning at the age of forty, or at thirty if there is a strong family history of cancer. Some of my patients express concern that over a period of time x-rays may *cause* cancer. It's true that very intensive exposure to radiation can do that. But in the case of x-rays of the breast, the irradiation is very small, and you have no cause for worry. Evidence around the world shows that mammography, even without clinical examination, reduces mortality from breast cancer among women over fifty by about 30 percent.

The mammogram is simply an x-ray of the breast.

Remember that the purpose of a mammogram is not to make a diagnosis. Only through microscopic examination of cells can we really know for certain whether a woman has breast cancer. The mammogram is rather a kind of screening. It helps us detect masses too small to be detected by the hand. Once they have been detected, only the microscopic examination of sample cells can tell us whether they are malignant.

What rouses our suspicions in a mammogram is no more than an irregular shadow with fuzzy margins or calcium deposits. To be sure, that's not much to go on. We make errors in interpretation in 15–20 percent of the cases. But mammograms are an essential part of the detection process. They can detect masses too small to be detected by hand.

Mammograms help detect masses too small to be detected by hand.

Where palpation or the mammogram raises a suspicion, biopsy must resolve it. I've had patients who out of fear did not take that next step and later died because the cancer had been allowed to spread, or metastasize. Please don't, out of fear or neglect, be one of their number.

THE BIOPSY

Up to this point, I've been talking about how we detect trouble signs. The biopsy, as you know, is strictly diagnostic. It tells us whether that trouble sign points to a malignancy. The happy fact is that the biopsy often points to some minor disorder, easily treatable.

Why, then, should you be subjected to this procedure when, in 80 percent of the cases, the results are negative? The answer is simple and urgent. An estimated 211,240 women will contract breast cancer in 2005. Among them, an estimated 40,410 will die, and of these, 5,640 will be African American. If these cancers were discovered early, through mammograms and biopsies, we might have prevented thousands of deaths per year.

Women worry about biopsy as a serious surgical procedure, and in the old days they had some reason to. For one thing, when our ability to interpret mammograms was less precise, biopsies were sometimes performed unnecessarily—in some cases because the radiologist feared a malpractice suit.

Now, happily, most surgeons proceed differently. Before the surgery, with the help of mammograms, the surgeon has a pretty clear idea of what has to be done. The patient learns the treatment plan in detail, and is free to make her decision. The surgeon doesn't move forward with-

In four cases out of five, the biopsy points to some minor disorder, easily treatable.

out her informed consent. Afterward, the treatment procedure is explained to family members.

In cases where, by palpation, I determine that the mass was a cyst (a fluid-filled mass), I remove all the fluid from the mass by a simple procedure called needle aspiration. Then the cyst collapses and disappears. In most cases, it does not recur. This procedure is done in my office. When the patient returns in a month for an exam, if the cyst *has* recurred, I repeat the procedure, again aspirating the cyst—that is, letting the fluid out. Only if it recurred a third time would I surgically remove the cyst.

If the mass proves to be solid and *not* to be a cyst, I get a sample of it by means of a biopsy. The pathology report will tell us whether cancer was present or not.

For patients who may not know the name of a doctor who can diagnose and treat them for cancer and who don't have a family doctor or HMO system that can refer them to one, the first step is to seek consultation at a breast cancer center. Typically, in such centers, a patient can have a mammogram, biopsy, surgery if necessary, and irradiation and chemotherapy done in one building. If you don't know where there is a center near you, call the National Institutes of Health's Cancer Information Service at (800) 4-CANCER. They'll refer you to a local treatment center.

THE ANATOMY AND PHYSIOLOGY
OF THE BREAST

Before I explain in more detail the kinds of treatments available to us and the types of cancer in which they're appropriate to use, I must first say something about the breast itself.

Obviously, to describe the breast simply in terms of its anatomy misses much of the point. Almost from the beginning of human time, the breast has gathered great cultural and symbolic significance. It has been an object of admiration, and sometimes even an object of terror.

For a woman, the breast is one expression of her beauty and womanhood. I have known patients who were devastated when the ligaments that support the breast became lax with several pregnancies or advancing age so that the once shapely breasts became "knee beaters." And I have known women to panic when they discover a "knot" in a breast while they are bathing, or as the result of a mammogram or ultrasound examination that points to cancer.

The breast is not an organ, like the heart or lung. Rather, it is a sweat gland that has been modified in the course of evolution. Its primary function is as a mammary gland that produces milk for the young. For that reason, it is made up of sacs, or small glands, where milk is produced, and ducts that carry the milk from the sacs to the nipple.

The female hormone, estrogen, stimulates cells through *estrogen receptors* in the lining of the sac and ducts. Too much estrogen can cause an abnormal growth in these cells and, eventually, a tumor that may be benign (noncancerous) or malignant (cancerous). A malignant tumor, left untreated, will eventually spread to other organs, such as the liver or lungs, using either the blood circulatory system or the lymphatic system as its avenues for movement into new areas.

TREATMENT

The treatment that a doctor recommends depends on the precise stage of the cancer. We classify cancers according to their severity,

FIGURE 3
ANATOMY OF THE BREAST

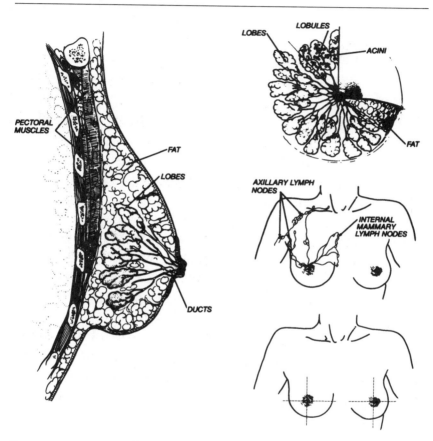

from stage 0 to stage IV. The principle here, as you'll see, is that the further the cancer has grown or spread, the higher the number.

- Stage 0 cancer we call *carcinoma in-situ.* This means that scattered cancerous cells have been detected, but they have not penetrated the floor of the tissue on which they rest. Removal of the tissue where these irregular sheets of cells occur will provide a complete cure.
- Stage I means that a tumor has formed but is confined to the breast and measures less than 2 cm in size. (One inch equals 2.2 centimeters.)

- Stage II means that (1) although the tumor is still less than 2 cm in size, it has spread to nodes in the armpit, or (2) the tumor is between 2 to 5 cm but has not spread to the armpit nodes.
- Stage III means that the tumor is larger than 5 cm in size or has many nodes in the armpit or has also invaded underlying muscle.
- Stage IV indicates that the cancer has spread to more distant parts of the body—like liver, lung, or bone.

STAGES 0–I

The earlier the stage of the cancer, the more options there are for treatment. Increasingly, we have veered away from modified radical mastectomy—that is, the removal of the entire breast—though in some cases it is necessary. Instead, where possible, we attack the cancer through *segmental resection* and *axillary sampling* for tumors—techniques that remove less tissue than a mastectomy does.

When the cancer is *in-situ,* that is, when it has not spread through the floor of tissue the cancer cells rest on, our procedure must depend in part on whether the cancer is lobular or ductal. Lobular cancer *in-situ* presents a particular problem. Although it is not frank, or invasive, cancer, it seems to be a predictor that the patient may develop cancer in both breasts. For this reason, when it is diagnosed, some surgeons recommend removal of both breasts.

The earlier the stage of the cancer, the more options there are for treatment.

I myself consider such an approach too drastic. I prefer to observe these patients carefully with mammograms and examinations twice a year. If frank cancer does develop, removal of both breasts may become necessary because this kind of cancer is associated with many tumors in both breasts.

Ductal cancer *in-situ* requires, in my judgment, total removal of the tumor with a rim of normal tissue, followed by radiation therapy.

In the case of either lobular or ductal cancers, a drug like tamoxifen can be effective in keeping the cancer from spreading. Some patients with these cancers may wish to enter clinical trials.

TREATMENT OF LOCALLY ADVANCED STAGE BREAST CANCERS

In stage II breast cancer, the tumor either has spread to the underarm or is larger than two inches in diameter. Lumpectomy or segmental resection, though they remain options, are riskier than they were at stage I. What I try to do for my own patients is to guide them by laying out the risks and benefits of each option. The patient herself must make the final decision.

In my own practice, I am not inclined to recommend lumpectomy or segmental resection in these cases. My reasoning is that because the cancer is advanced, the risk of recurrent or persistent cancer would be too high.

Women fifty years old or younger often opt for a *segmentectomy*, meaning that a quarter of the breast is removed, with chemotherapy and radiation to follow. In such cases, I have them consult with a radiologist beforehand because in a large breast x-rays may not penetrate deeply enough; and in a small one, a shrunken, fibrotic and painful breast can result.

Modified radical mastectomy is, in my judgment, often the better course. This means removing the breast along with underarm tissue, thus removing all local lymph nodes.

I don't take lightly the emotional cost mastectomy imposes on a woman. But this procedure gives more insurance than the others that we have removed all tumors on the chest wall and underarm. Followed by some combination of chemotherapy, radiation, and hormonal drugs, it often proves effective.

Stage III cancers reduce the options still further. Here, the cancer has spread but has not gone into distant organs. Where the cancer isn't of the *inflammatory* type—the breast swollen and hot, the skin of the breast broken out in a rash that may give it the appearance of an orange peel—it can sometimes be treated successfully with a modified mastectomy. Often, at this stage, the cancer *has* spread, but it has not yet reached distant organs.

Patients may choose not to submit to a mastectomy at this point. When they do, if the tumor has begun to ulcerate, I strongly recommend at least a *total mastectomy*. If this procedure is followed by hormonal therapy and chemotherapy, it is sometimes successful.

When inflammatory cancer *does* appear, a patient may think that it is an infection. But because an apparent infection *can* prove to be cancer, it is essential that the patient have it examined at once. Any delay will increase the danger.

The inflammatory type of breast cancer is obviously very dangerous. Radical surgery at this stage isn't appropriate. It does no good. Instead, treatment takes the form of irradiation, hormonal therapy, and chemotherapy. The patient's chances of survival are poor once the cancer has reached this stage.

TREATMENT OF ADVANCED OR RECURRENT STAGE BREAST CANCER

Stage IV breast cancer means that the cancer has spread, or metastasized, to distant sites or organs. The likely organs to be affected are the lung, liver, brain, bone, ovary, or skin. The approach to stage IV cancer is palliative, meaning that improving the quality of the patient's life and or survival duration is the goal, rather than curing the patient. Since the tumor has become systemic, or spread well beyond the breast, local therapies like surgeries are ineffective in terms of cure. Hence, systemic treatment in the form of chemotherapy or palliative radiation therapy can be effective in prolonging the patient's life for sometimes up to seven years. In some circumstances, these methods may potentially shrink or delay tumor growth, thereby increasing the patient's survival and perhaps improving his/her quality of life. Some stage IV breast cancer patients are able to lead relatively active lives while undergoing regular treatment.

A stage IV breast cancer diagnosis should not be seen as a hopeless finality. With the constant advent of new research and clinical trials, physicians and health care providers are sometimes able to extend and improve a patient's life in even advanced stages of breast cancer. Many stage IV breast cancer survivors have found that living with serious illness even gives them a new perspective on life. Some patients find that they are able to embrace what is truly important to them and discard trivial concerns that clouded their lives before receiving their diagnosis. Reaching out in support groups to other survivors and realizing that they are not on a frightening journey alone can create friendships that help them endure. There is a quote that is often heard in these groups: "Healing is not a cure." This idea of inner healing often inspires stage IV breast cancer survivors to find balance, connectedness, and peace not dependent on medicine, but rather within themselves.

MASTECTOMY AND SELF-IMAGE

For women and men alike, one's sense of self depends in part on body image. Mastectomy in any form threatens a woman's self-image. To lose what makes one attractive, in one's own eyes and the eyes of others, threatens one's sense of self. But most women work this through by keeping one thing very clear. The choice is between personal vanity and one's life. Although the first is unquestionably important, few of us would willingly buy it at the expense of our lives.

You'll want to talk with other women who have been through this surgery. You'll find that most of them are doing quite nicely. Happily, the human spirit is most resourceful, and as I'll show you further in later chapters, many people come out of such experience stronger than they were when they went in.

ADJUVANT THERAPY

Adjuvant therapy refers to any therapy that is used in addition to primary therapy (usually surgery) for breast cancer. Adjuvant therapy can be used before surgery (neoadjuvant therapy) or after surgery (adjuvant therapy). It is usually categorized as either systemic or localized. Systemic adjuvant therapy means that the treatment's focus is on the whole body whereas localized adjuvant therapy means that the focus is on the tumor. Systemic adjuvant therapy includes chemotherapy and hormone therapy; radiation therapy is considered localized adjuvant treatment. Oncologists (doctors who specialize in the treatment of cancer) might start a patient on a single type, or combination, of adjuvant therapies before surgery because often this approach will reduce the size of the mass and therefore make it somewhat easier to resect. This, in turn, helps decrease the chance of the tumor's recurrence. It is important to remember that each patient's treatment will be based on a variety of factors unique to him/her. No one method works for everyone, and several prognostic and predictive factors will be taken into account when determining whether or not adjuvant therapy will be necessary.

Let's now look at some of the different types of adjuvant therapy.

RADIATION

The purpose of radiation therapy is to kill the cancer cells. The radiation is commonly administered through a large x-ray machine. Radioactive material can also be placed directly into the breast through small plastic tubes.

Such treatments are time consuming and hard on the patient. Radiation treatments tend to be a full-time job: they require that the patient visit the clinic five days a week for six weeks.

Such treatments can be hard on older women, or women with other health problems. Transportation can also be a problem. Not everyone has an easy way to get to the hospital and back five days a week. And if others depend on them, women may find it difficult to give that much time to their cure.

Radiation may cause pain or ulcers in the breast, or make the breasts lose their suppleness or even to become hard. These effects can be similar to those that accompany an intense sunburn. Patients may find it uncomfortable to wear a bra.

In earlier times, it wasn't uncommon for excessively high doses of radiation to be given. These could result in inflammation and scarring in the lung, with accompanying shortness of breath. Nowadays, such problems are rare. But even with today's more precise techniques, some damage to normal structures can occur, as we will describe in the section on complications.

Except to treat cancers of the mouth, cervix, or prostate, radiation treatment is rarely if ever a primary treatment. It is usually given for the purpose of relieving pain and slowing metastases, where radiation *can* be a primary means of cure. Sometimes its potential effectiveness for slowing the growth of the cancer can be helpful before surgery. Its role here is to shrink the cancer mass so that surgery can be done on a smaller area. Used with lumpectomy or segmentectomy, radiation treatment with chemotherapy can be very effective.

Given the complications and difficulties of radiation therapy, a patient must be prepared in advance for it. That preparation is her responsibility in that she or her loved ones must put the right questions to the doctor. By knowing what to expect, and by consciously choosing it, a patient will be emotionally prepared for the treatment. The last thing a patient needs is unnecessary surprises.

QUESTIONS FOR YOUR DOCTOR

Doctors can seem very busy, and often they are. But it's not your job to worry about that. Their business is their problem. Your problem is cancer. And you're going to have a better chance of cure if you understand your treatment.

- Your understanding ensures that you'll decide on a surgical treatment as early as possible, knowing that long delays can endanger your life.
- Your understanding ensures that you won't miss appointments for x-ray or chemotherapy treatment.
- Your understanding ensures that you will report to your doctor any sign that the cancer has returned.
- Your understanding may also mean that you have invested your *will* in your cure, and I have known cases in which the human will itself proved a powerful medicine.

Don't be shy about asking questions. Patients sometimes feel they don't know enough to ask questions. You know enough. You simply need to prepare. Write your questions down before you visit your doctor, and don't be ashamed to take the paper out and read from it. The sorts of questions you might want to ask are these:

- When does the treatment begin and end?
- How long will each treatment last?
- How often must I be at the clinic each week?
- How long will each treatment last?
- Exactly how does this irradiation work? And how are you going to get it into me?
- What will be its effects on my body? I want to hear the bad ones along with the good ones.
- Might I get sick enough from irradiation to have to stay in the hospital?
- Even if I don't get sick, will I be well enough to go to work and take care of my kids?
- Will the treatment make my breast insensitive?
- How good are the chances that this treatment will cure me?
- What are the chances that the cure will be permanent?
- Can I still have plastic surgery in the area if the radiation affects underlying tissue and healing?

You'll naturally have many more questions of your own to add to this list. Don't be afraid to ask them. Tell the doctor in advance that you are going to want a reasonably big piece of his or her time. Your doctor will understand you. It's your life that's under discussion, so you must do what you can to ensure that the discussion is generous and clear.

After a surgical procedure or biopsy, the tissue that has been taken is examined under a microscope by a pathologist, one who studies human tissues on a cellular level. Using a microscope, the pathologist is able to determine whether the cells in the examined tissue are normal. If they demonstrate cancerous changes, they are classified as either *in situ*, not growing beyond certain boundaries, or invasive, which means these cancer cells have extended beyond normal membranes. Once a tumor has been identified, it is measured. The size of the tumor becomes very important in prognosis and treatment regimens. Next, the specimen is examined to evaluate whether or not the tumor extends to the edge of the specimen, or the margin. In those circumstances where the tumor involves the margin, it is immediately suspected that some of the tumor has been left behind in the body. Further surgery may then be warranted.

Breast cancer tumor cells typically spread through the lymphatic system, into the local/regional lymph nodes. As a result, lymph nodes are often evaluated for tumor spread by the pathologist. Those patients with lymphatic involvement have a prognosis that is inversely proportional to the number of nodes involved. A pathologist might also describe the tumor by its grade. The grade measures how aggressive or abnormal the cancer cells are compared to normal cells.

There are three important tests that can be performed to assess a patient's prognosis. As we previously discussed, certain breast cancer cells grow with the help of estrogen receptors (ER) and progesterone receptors (PR). Not all patients will demonstrate this type of cancer, however, so whether or not they are positive will determine if they will be receptive to hormone therapy. They are usually categorized as ER+/ER-, and PR+/PR-. Additionally, if a patient tests positive for Human Epithelial Receptor 2 Neu (HER2neu) gene, his/her cancer tends to be more aggressive. Further tests like the MRI and PET/CT SCAN can be helpful as supportive diagnostic tools in cancer detection and in giving information about the cancer's spread.

HORMONE THERAPY

The cancer cells for some women with breast cancer contain receptors like little cups, where the female hormones, estrogen and progesterone, are stored. With the help of these hormones, cancer cells can grow and spread. The object of hormone therapy in breast cancer is to reduce the exposure of the receptors to the female hormones. This can be accomplished with two types of medication: 1) tamoxifen, which blocks the receptor and prevents the cups from filling and 2) aromatase inhibitors, which can cause a decrease in the production of the female hormone. Both these agents are given orally.

Like most medications that have a powerful physiological impact, these hormone treatments (aromatase inhibitors) can have negative side effects. They can often weaken one's bones and perhaps lead to osteoporosis, increase cholesterol levels, raise the risk of blood clots, and cause upset stomach.

CHEMOTHERAPY

What Is Chemotherapy?

Chemotherapy refers to any of a group of medications that interfere with the function of the cancer cells to grow and that eventually causes them to die. These medicines may be given prior to surgery. Given before surgery, chemotherapy is known as "neoadjuvant"; after surgery it is called "adjuvant" therapy.

Why Give Chemotherapy?

Chemotherapy may be given prior to surgery to help reduce the size of a tumor mass. After surgery, chemotherapy helps keep the cancer from reoccurring. Chemotherapy may also be given to help relieve the symptoms of advanced cancer.

Who Gets Chemotherapy?

The doctor's decision to use a particular kind of chemotherapy is based on successful clinic investigations of this treatment on patients with symptoms and medical signs like yours. That benefit may be in keeping the tumor from recurring, make the tumor more amenable to surgery, and/or in relieving symptoms.

How Is Chemotherapy Given?

Chemotherapy is usually given intravenously, but it can also be given orally. Multidrug regimens of chemotherapy are usually given, usually on an outpatient basis, one day of treatment scheduled every two to four weeks. Such a cycle allows the patient's blood counts to recover enough to tolerate another round of chemo. Other chemo regimens are given over several days, often on an inpatient basis at your local hospital. If, after treatment and recovery time, your blood count isn't in a safe range, your doctor may delay treatment for one or two weeks until they *have* recovered. Such delays don't reduce the effectiveness of the treatment. In fact, the delays help to get the patient stronger and back on his or her feet.

An example of new oral chemo medications is the drug capecitabine (Xeloda®), an oral drug sometimes substituted in some treatment programs for 5-fluorouracil in the treatment of breast and colon cancers.

Xeloda® is an oral chemo medication you can take at home, under your doctor's frequent and careful supervision, and it is therefore convenient for those who can't get to hospitals easily because they live in remote areas or have hectic lifestyles. Xeloda®

has proven effective against metastatic breast cancer, metastatic colorectal cancer, and adjuvant colorectal cancer.

What Are the Side Effects of Chemotherapy?

The side effects from chemotherapy occur because the therapy does not distinguish between cancer cells and noncancer cells. For the brief period when needed healthy cells don't function, the patient may experience nausea, vomiting, decreased appetite, anemia, and infection.

The control of nausea and vomiting has changed dramatically with the addition of the serotonin antagonists. These drugs are ondansetron (Zofran®), granisetron (Kytril®), and dolasetron (Anzemet®) They have been proven effective and safe.

What Are Targeted Therapies?

Our knowledge of how cancer cells function has grown greatly over the past decades, and new knowledge has led to new kinds of treatment through agents that attack cancer in very specific areas.

QUESTIONS FOR YOUR DOCTOR

The patient owes it to herself to understand her chemotherapy treatment clearly in advance. To do that, there's no substitute for asking questions of your chemotherapist.

- How often must I come in for treatment?
- How long will each treatment take?
- Will I be able to drive myself home from treatment?
- What chemicals will you use, and what are their advantages and disadvantages?
- How ill from side effects of the drugs will I be during the course of treatment?
- When will you know if the treatments are effective?

CONTROLLING ESTROGEN WITH
TAMOXIFEN OR RALOXIFENE

For nearly twenty years, I have treated women who have breast cancer with a drug known as *tamoxifen*. It has proven effective in keeping the cancer from spreading and in reducing the recurrence of malignancy—that is, in keeping the cancerous condition from returning after treatment.

My own experience is confirmed by studies performed by the Breast Cancer Prevention Trial (funded by the National Cancer Institute). This large-scale human trial showed that invasive cancer—that is, cancer in stages I through III—was reduced by 49 percent in women who were on tamoxifen.

Unfortunately, tamoxifen, like many drugs, has undesirable side effects—specifically, it may cause cancer of the uterus. It may also cause blood clots in the legs, clots that can become dangerous if they move to other organs like the lungs.

Serious illness may require treatments that carry their own risks. There's no way around that. But researchers work steadily to reduce those risks. In the case of estrogen treatment, they've developed a new, related drug, *raloxifene*, that shows great promise in clinical trials. Raloxifene—like tamoxifen, a "designer hormone"— appears *not* to carry the danger of uterine cancer, and it has the further advantage of preventing osteoporosis (weak bones caused by lack of calcium). Though raloxifene, like tamoxifen, appears to cause blood clots, I urge African-American women to take part in clinical trials for this new drug. The benefits of this drug for women who have breast cancer far outweigh the drawbacks.

Currently, researchers are comparing the risks and benefits of these two drugs. The study called Study of tamoxifen and raloxifene (STAR) has recently published initial results showing that the drug raloxifene shows statistically equivalent reduction in invasive breast cancer. However, because raloxifene was originally a medication prescribed for post-menopausal women at risk for osteoporosis, it has the added benefit of protecting bone health. Yet tamoxifen puts breast cancer patients at risk for bone loss. Furthermore, raloxifene patients demonstrated fewer deep vein thromboses and fewer pulmonary embolisms, as well as fewer incidences of uterine cancer. Additionally, the initial results from STAR suggest that raloxifene does not increase the risk of developing a cataract, as tamoxifen does.

OTHER MEDICAL THERAPIES

So far, I've talked about the most common treatments for breast cancer—surgery, radiation, and chemotherapy—that, to the moment, have stood the test of time. However, other treatments are available.

Gene Therapy

You may have read that researchers have made a preliminary map of all of our genes. This is a very great achievement, whose implications we are only starting to imagine. Once the map is complete, we should be able to make exact diagnoses of all diseases, including cancer. And the possibilities don't end there. We may be able to manipulate the genes, correcting defects, eliminating diseased cells, and thus curing the patient.

At the moment, we are still at the early stages of what we call *gene therapy*. Because the treatment is novel, new dangers occur; and until these problems are worked out, progress in this area may be slow. But doctors involved in such research expect that within the next decade, such therapies will be in general use.

Immunotherapy

Another kind of therapy that doctors are experimenting with is called immunotherapy, also referred to as biological therapy. The principle behind immunotherapy is to use the body's own defense system, the immune system, to help fight or at least lessen the effects of cancer. Some biological therapies help the body to recognize cancer cells, prevent their spread, or even "reprogram" them to behave like normal cells. Hence, there are many different types of vaccines and treatments that enhance the body's own way of fighting the cancer cells. Currently, researchers are studying ways to use antibodies to specifically attack the receptors on cancer cells. One such important antibody in the treatment of breast cancer is Herceptin (trastuzumab). As we mentioned previously, some types of breast cancer are categorized according to different receptors for which they test positive. Patients who are considered HER2+ possess a gene which codes for a specific receptor on their cancer cells, the HER2 receptor which aids in the growth of these cancer cells. Herceptin targets these HER2 receptors on cancer cells, thereby incapacitating the cell's ability to grow.

Because there are many different factors that help a tumor grow, there are many different philosophies on how it can be stopped. Just like normal, healthy cells, cancerous cells require a blood supply in order to grow. A tumor creates a tiny network of blood vessels, known as capillaries, around itself so that it may extend and grow. In order to do this, it uses a protein called vascular endothelial growth factor (VEGF) to help create its web. However, an antibody called Avastin (Bevacizumab) attaches itself to this protein, thus inhibiting the cancer cell's ability to grow.

COMPLICATIONS THAT MAY FOLLOW TREATMENT

Cancer treatment involves strong medicine, including surgery. Strong medicines sometimes mean complications, or problems that result from the treatment itself. Let me guide you through some of these complications.

Complications That May Follow Mastectomy
Though I have performed several hundred breast operations, I have never lost a single patient as a result of the surgery itself. For this, I am grateful to the excellent anesthesiologists I have worked with. Whenever general anesthesia is used, serious heart and lung prob-

lems can occur. But a good anesthesiologist knows how to use the least amount of anesthesia necessary to guarantee that the patient will experience no pain.

Naturally, patients worry about the wound itself. We all know that in the case of any cuts, infections can develop during the healing period. In surgery, however, because the wound is clean and carefully treated, infection is rare. If the tumor that has been removed has ulcerated, there is more danger of infection. But because we anticipate that danger and prepare against it, it rarely occurs.

One postoperative problem that *can* occur is that the skin around the scar may slough off. This can happen if the surgeon pulls the skin together too tightly while he or she is attempting to close the wound, thereby accidentally cutting off the blood supply to the skin. If sloughing occurs, skin grafting may be necessary in order to close the wound.

Swelling of the arm after axillary dissection occurs in some cases. This happens if the normal movement of fluid called *lymphatic fluid* has been interrupted either by the tumor itself or by scarring from surgery. The lymphatic fluid normally is drained to the lymph glands in the armpit. When these glands are removed, fluid backs up into the arm and swelling (*lymphedema*) results.

The problem can be caused, or aggravated, by irradiation to the axilla after dissection, so we try to avoid that combination of treatments. The condition can be relieved through physical therapy.

Finally, the scar left behind from surgery may become fibrotic and hard. That condition, called a *keloid*, is especially common in blacks. We can help relieve the condition by injecting cortisone, and also by applying cocoa butter or vitamin E cream to the scar. But burning and itching where a keloid has developed can continue for some time.

Complications That May Follow Irradiation

Radiation therapy can cause problems of its own, and should always be used cautiously. In certain cases, it should not be used at all. This is true in the case of patients who suffer from diseases like lupus and scleroderma. It is also true of patients who have already received x-ray treatment to the chest wall, or patients who are pregnant. Because irradiation can damage the heart and lungs, we must be especially cautious about treatment in those areas. Finally, we must take special care in treating with radiation small breasts from which a tumor has been removed by conservative surgery. Because if the breasts are exposed to too much radiation, they may become shrunken, hardened, fibrotic, and painful. The cosmetic result is then poor.

Radiation can also cause the skin to become burned and to blister. The ribs can be damaged so that they become easily fractured.

Complications That May Follow Chemotherapy

Chemotherapy is toxic. It frequently causes nausea, diarrhea, and vomiting. It often causes hair loss though that corrects itself after the therapy is complete.

As bad as these are, there can be still more serious side effects of chemotherapy. One of the most dreaded of these is suppression, or weakening, of your bone marrow. Since the bone marrow is crucial to the immune system, if it isn't working well you become more susceptible to disease and infection.

We are having some success in controlling bone marrow suppression by transplanting healthy marrow to replace what's damaged. We can also give proteins that stimulate the growth of immune cells. Strengthening the immune system in these ways allows us to use chemotherapy more aggressively, knowing that we can control this negative effect.

Particular drugs carry particular risks. The drug doxorubicin, often used in chemotherapy, may cause heart problems.

Methotrexate can cause pneumonitis, an inflammation of the lung that, unlike pneumonia itself, may result from other causes than bacteria. Methotrexate may also cause bleeding from the intestinal lining and destruction of the liver.

Remember that these side effects are *uncommon*. If you read the manufacturer's information sheet on almost *any* drug, you'll find that, on rare occasions, it may cause terrible side effects. Not only are the severe symptoms extremely rare, but in most cases stopping use of the drug that causes the symptoms will reverse them.

Complications That May Follow Hormonal Treatment

Hormonal therapy is, strictly speaking, not toxic, but it too has its dangers. Tamoxifen, for example, which lowers estrogen levels in the breast, also affects the estrogen in the uterus and may cause uterine cancer. Hormonal therapy can sometimes cause blood clots in the legs, which can become dangerous if they move to the lungs.

But these negative effects are relatively rare. Since many women who used the drug experienced improvement, we must consider the side effects necessary evils if they occur.

It isn't easy to balance benefits and risks in these matters. It takes great courage to begin a therapy that you know may carry dangers of its own. That's why it's important for you to have informed conversations with your physician about the best therapy for you. Only you can decide what risks, and, yes, what suffering, you are prepared to take for the sake of a cure.

But however you resolve these questions, one fact must remain clear: delaying therapy or putting it off altogether has to be your worst choice. The key to curing cancer is early diagnosis and early effective treatment.

REHABILITATION

Rehabilitation from any major disease is a hard job, and it can be a long one. It requires of the patient great investment, both physical and emotional. Fortunately, the patient isn't in this alone. Rehabilitation needs the help of a team that can work together as one—a team made up of the patient, the family, and the health care staff.

If you're the patient, you may want to ask a loved one or friend to help organize that team. It will be the team's job, as well as yours, to know beforehand as much as it can about the stages of recovery. The more you and your team know, the better prepared you can be.

Even if you live alone, your doctor or social worker can help you get in touch with support groups that can assist you through the post-operative stage. (One of these, called Reach to Recovery, a program organized by women, I know to be very helpful. But there are many other good groups, and they're easy to find.) No matter how strong you are, rehabilitation is not a job you'll want to do alone. You need people to talk to, people to help you keep your spirits up when they sag.

A positive mental attitude is essential to your recovery. Without that, the return to normal life is difficult at best, and in the worst cases, it becomes impossible. I know a woman who lived alone but would not contact a recovery group. After surgery, she plunged into a depression that became disabling. She could not bring herself to my office for a checkup, or to the hospital for follow-up treatment, nor would she receive visitors or even perform the necessary reha-bilitation exercises. Fear, depression, and self-imposed isolation pre-vented her from making a full recovery. In effect, that first bout of breast cancer destroyed her life—because she let it.

I don't make light of the courage it takes to come back from a bout of a disease as serious as breast cancer. But most patients, with the help of people who love them, rise to that challenge. For many patients, recovery and healing leaves them stronger than they were before.

It is very important—indeed, *essential*—that husbands, family, and loved ones let the patient know early and steadily that a mas-tectomy has in no sense diminished her value as a woman or as a human being. The patient will need reassurance. Even a negative glance may kindle her own fear that with the loss of a breast, or even a less radical operation, she has lost what makes her a woman. For the patient, there's an intimate connection between self-esteem and the esteem granted by others. A smile, a touch of the hand, can tip the balance toward a healthy emotional state and recovery.

For a married woman, the husband's support is obviously most important. The worst-case scenario, one that I actually witnessed firsthand, is a husband who simply turns his back on his recovering wife. This particular husband, whom, as a man, I remember with shame, never visited his wife after her operation. When she returned home, he had moved out of the house. You can imagine the effect of this on a woman who has just gone through serious surgery and who is struggling with her own doubts.

What that man did made him less than a man. In a situation like this, family members must look beyond the tips of their own noses. They must see and respond to the patient's need. They must understand the patient's anger or depression. In these cases, the husband, the family, a friend, the minister, and church members all must play a part.

This, too, is a moment when the doctor and the office staff must also be compassionate. It's their job to help relieve the pain, both psychological and physical. It's their job to return promptly phone calls from the patient or her loved ones and to give a sympathetic ear and professional advice.

I've taken a lot of time over this subject because it's a critical one. Nothing is more important for the patient's ongoing health than her mental state in the first weeks after surgery. If she is calm and determined, and confident of the love around her, she'll turn easily to the rehabilitative exercises she needs to perform regularly. Through these exercises, she will regain strength and mobility of shoulder, arm, and hand. The exercise must begin just a few days after the surgery. Once a regular exercise routine is established, the patient will be heartened to feel the pain and stiffness vanishing.

Patience, determination, and steadiness are the essential prescriptions for recovery. A woman who has been well all of her life may not find it easy to schedule and appear for the many necessary followup visits to the physician and surgeon. The better the patient understands the disease, the better the motivation.

Examinations will be necessary throughout the patient's life. Once a year, she will need a complete physical exam that includes careful attention to the chest wall, axilla, the other breast, neck, lungs, and abdomen. She will also need annual mammograms.

The examining doctor will give very careful attention to the opposite breast from the one in which the cancer appeared and was treated. The patient herself will also want to give careful and regular attention to it, and to report to her doctor any noted changes. Such vigilance can be emotionally trying, and each woman must work out a way that allows her to be careful without being panicky. Here, the help of other women who have been through these stages before is invaluable.

The patient will need to pay attention to the overall state of her body. In ordinary life, we're sometimes too busy to pay much attention to how we feel. But the recovering cancer patient *must* be ready to mark any unusual pain or symptoms—especially the following:

- New pain
- Weight loss
- Decrease of appetite
- Weakness
- Coughing
- Changes in the menstrual cycle.

These can be early warning signs of metastases—that is, spreading—of the cancer. Often, these metastases can be controlled by hormonal therapy or chemotherapy.

Yes, the recovering patient requires patience—that's what the word "patient" means, after all—in adjusting to her therapeutic routines and checkups. But as important as that is, it's equally important that she return to normal life and all of her previous activities as early as possible. Yes, return to work. Go to church or to club meetings. Participate in family and other social activities. Learn to enjoy again all the things you enjoyed before.

It's the nature of some people to keep their personal anxieties and disturbances to themselves. But a recovering cancer patient is entitled to share her moments of doubt and fear with others. Talk to friends about your concerns. Only if you articulate those fears can others help you. And be willing to talk with your husband about sexual matters. If he is a man, and a real husband, he will know how to soothe your fears.

Finally, though we *can* look at statistics and gauge our chances against the outcomes of similar cases, each case is different from all others. Just as each of us has a unique personality and emotional makeup, so each has a highly individual genetic and psychological makeup, including a unique set of immune responses. Only your doctor, who knows the most about your individual makeup and medical history, can advise you about your particular situation and probable outcome.

But even your doctor may, in the end, be a less accurate predictor than you. It's the patient alone who knows her will to live, her appetite for life, her confidence in the power of love in her and around her. The secret, as I know from my own experience, is to live each day to its fullest, with no regrets for yesterday and prayerful hope for tomorrow.

For more on the important subject of rehabilitation, see Chapters 22–24. I also recommend that you look at the National Cancer Institute's Web site, at *www.cancer.gov*. You'll find a vast amount of useful information there on cancer prevention, screening, and supportive care.

WHY CANCER RUNS IN FAMILIES

If breast cancer runs in your family, it may be the result of inherited damaged genes. In this case, those genes become a risk factor for you. Their presence indicates that you are more likely to get breast cancer.

When mutations of these genes appear in women (and they do in only 1 percent of the population), women are three to seven times more likely to develop breast cancer than women without alterations in these genes. Women with these altered genes may also have a higher risk for colon cancer. Some women with a strong family history of breast cancer opt for bilateral breast mastectomy—that is, the removal of both breasts. Such a surgical operation is a strong insurance policy against developing breast cancer, but it is not a foolproof one. A small percentage of women may suffer recurrence of cancer after the operation.

When mutations of these genes appear in men, they too have a higher risk for breast cancer, and possibly of prostate cancer as well. Investigations to determine whether the mutations contribute to other cancers as well are ongoing.

PROGNOSIS

The word *prognosis* means prediction. The difficulty with most predictions is that there are too many variables to take into account, and that, like everything in nature, these variables change even as we try to identify them. That's why weather forecasters miss the mark so often. And that's why your doctor can miss the mark, too.

In the case of breast cancer, or any cancer for that matter, accurate prognosis depends on identifying the *stage* of the cancer and providing adequate treatment. We've already seen that because of the seriousness of the disease, the way cancer spreads in the body, the difficulty of eliminating every trace of it, and the toxic effect of some of the treatments themselves, cancer treatment is both risky and potentially dangerous.

Let me be honest with you and say that predicting the outcome of a cancer and assuring a good outcome are also risky. The reasons why this is so I can illustrate best by example.

Let's assume that a breast cancer patient has opted for modified radical mastectomy. The advantage of that procedure is that it offers the best chance of removing every piece of fat and every lymph node in the armpit, including removal of the breast itself, which is the original site of the cancer. But practical considerations prevent us from dissecting and examining under the microscope *every* bit of tissue that we have removed.

For us to identify the exact stage of a cancer, we would need to remove and examine *every* lymph node. This is nearly impossible. But even if it were possible, there would remain much room for error.

FIGURE 4

BREAST CANCER INCIDENCE RATES, 1975–2002
by Age, *In-Situ* Versus Malignant All Races, Female

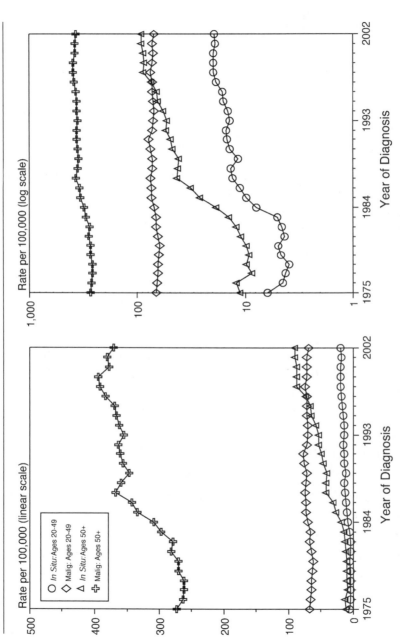

Legend:
- ○ *In Situ:* Ages 20-49
- ◇ Malig: Ages 20-49
- △ *In Situ:* Ages 50+
- ☩ Malig: Ages 50+

Year of Diagnosis

Rate per 100,000 (linear scale)

Rate per 100,000 (log scale)

Year of Diagnosis

Source: SEER 9 areas. Rates are age-adjusted to the 2000 US Std Population (19 age groups - Census P25-1103).

Surveillance, Epidemiology, and End Results (SEER) Program (www.seer.cancer.gov) SEER*Stat Database: Incidence - SEER 9 Regs Public-Use, Nov 2004 Sub (1973-2002), National Cancer Institute, DCCPS, Surveillance Research Program, Cancer Statistics Branch, released April 2005, based on the November 2004 submission

FIGURE 5

BREAST CANCER INCIDENCE AND MORTALITY, 1975–2002
White Females Versus Black Females

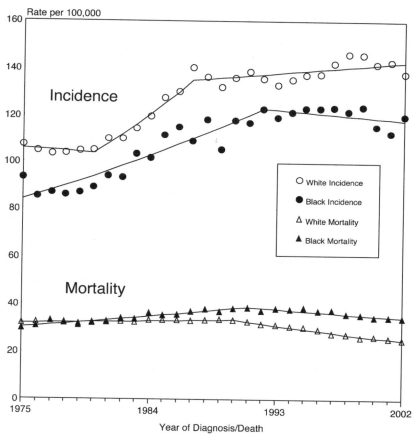

Source: SEER 9 areas and NCHS public use data file for the total US.
Rates are age-adjusted to the 2000 US Std Population (19 age groups - Census P25-1103).
Regression lines are calculated using the Joinpoint Regression Program Version 3.0, April 2005, National Cancer Institute.

Surveillance, Epidemiology, and End Results (SEER) Program (www.seer.cancer.gov) SEER*Stat Database: Incidence - SEER 9 Regs Public-Use, Nov 2004 Sub (1973-2002), National Cancer Institute, DCCPS, Surveillance Research Program, Cancer Statistics Branch, released April 2005, based on the November 2004 submission.

The upshot is that doctors and clinicians are scientists, but we are also human. And to be human is to be imperfect—that is, to be confined by limits of judgment, execution, and technology. Our techniques and equipment will improve, and so will the kinds of treatment available to us. But perfection is an attribute that belongs to God alone, not to human beings.

Having said all that, I can tell you the good news. Stage I and stage II cancer patients treated by mastectomy, whether radical or modified, with the help of postsurgical therapy, have a 71 to 78 percent chance of being cancer-free at the end of five years. Seventy-five percent of such patients who are alive at the end of five years will also be alive at the end of ten years. These good figures underline the necessity of early diagnosis. If we can catch the cancer early enough, you have a very good chance to recover completely.

Many mysteries remain in our search for how cancer comes and goes, why it shows itself at one time and hides itself at another. I have known cases where a patient has appeared cancer-free for fifteen years, only for the cancer then to occur in distant organs. Such cases are not common, but they happen. The question they raise is: where was the cancer in the interval?

We believe that in such cases the immune system may have held the cancer in check. So one of our aims is to find ways to strengthen the immune system and to help our patients avoid doing anything that might weaken it. You can find out more about strengthening the immune system in Chapter 3, on diet and prevention.

RECONSTRUCTION

Only a woman can know what it means to be told she must lose one of her breasts, or even both of them. Her womanhood, her beauty, her very sense of herself—all are threatened at once. The fact is most women can reconcile themselves to the physical loss when they understand how urgent it is to their survival. I don't wish to pretend that it isn't a terrible loss. But what helps and matters to some extent is that the plastic surgeon can make a new breast to replace the old. In some cases, the plastic surgery is done at the same time as the mastectomy itself.

The surgical procedure is relatively simple. The surgeon frees up the muscles that lie beneath the breast and inserts a saline bag there. As an alternative, the surgeon will in some cases fill the defect left in the chest wall with a muscle from the back or with fat from the abdomen.

Mastectomy, like any surgical procedure, can lead to complications. Sometimes—and this is rare—skin loss or infections in the implant area may result. Further, certain kinds of reconstructive surgery can make it more difficult to detect the cancer should it return. But these days, because we place the implant under the muscles, recurrence is less of a problem than it once was.

IN A NUTSHELL

Incidence:
The incidence of breast cancer is 143.2 per 100,000 for white women, and 118.6 per 100,000 among black women. Mortality rates are 26.4 per 100,000 for white women, and 35.4 per 100,000 for black women. Indeed, the mortality rate for African Americans is the highest of all races surveyed. That's not a record to be admired.

Cause:
Specific causes are unknown, but are thought to include:
- Genetic makeup
- Lifestyle and diet
- Breast receptors stimulated by estrogen
- Environmental factors

Prevention:
Decrease estrogen effect on breast by:
- Eating a low-fat diet rich in fruits, vegetables, fish, fiber, soy

- Stopping smoking
- Exercising regularly
- Taking tamoxifen or raloxifene.

Diagnosis:
The three-point play:
- Monthly self-examination from age of twenty
- Yearly mammogram from age of forty
- Clinical exam yearly from age of forty.

Treatment:
Early treatment includes:
- Lumpectomy and x-ray
- Chemotherapy
- Modified radical mastectomy
- Clinical trial.

Prognosis:
Stages I and II, excellent to good
Stage III, fair
Stage IV, poor

SIX

Colon Cancer

EVEN THE PATH TO A diagnosis of cancer of the colon had meant for Jack a period of uncertainty and anxiety. It was as if he had been suddenly dropped into a foreign country whose language was just noise to him.

When the doctor first examined Jack, he spoke of the possibility of an ulcer. Then, after Jack had been given more tests, the doctor spoke of "a mass," "a polyp," "a malignancy," and, finally, "a cancer." For Jack, it was as if a net (or, he sometimes thought, a noose) was being tightened around him. He had hoped against hope that they'd settle on a less threatening diagnosis—he *hoped* it would turn out to be an ulcer. But as test results began to come in, the verdict became inescapable.

At first, Jack refused to give attention to the details of his illness. He'd proudly avoided doctors all his life. Now it made him nervous when, in the examination rooms, his wife Anna asked question after question. How reliable was the diagnosis? What were the treatment options? What were the advantages and the disadvantages of each?

Jack would sit there uneasily, feeling worse and worse as she kept up her flow of questions, even taking notes. Back home, he'd tell her:

"Anna, I know you're trying to help, but all this talk just makes things worse for me. The doctors know what they're doing; let's just let 'em do it. I just want to get this over with."

But Anna persisted, reading books, talking to people. She learned a lot about how doctors thought about colon cancer, about the terminology, and about possible treatment plans. After the first few days, Jack came around and began to learn with her.

"Listen to me, honey," she said to him the day after they'd decided on surgery. "If we'd understood more about this a year, or even six months, ago, we'd have got you diagnosed a lot earlier. Those minor complaints you were having back then could have given us a clue.

"Now we're going to learn what we can about your recovery and follow-up treatment. You're going to be the best patient these doctors have ever seen, and they're going to give you their best. And I'm going to keep you with me for a long time, what do you think about that?"

Jack couldn't find much here to argue with. Who can argue against love? Even before he went to the hospital for his surgery, he knew a lot about what to expect, and a lot about what he'd have to do to recuperate. He felt ready. This would be the biggest struggle of his life, but he felt prepared for it, and his last thought before he went under the anesthesia was how sweet it would be in a week or so to take his first postoperative walk around their block.

FACTS ABOUT COLORECTAL CANCER

Colon and rectal cancer, often referred to as "colorectal," are the third most common cancers in males and the second most common in females. In 2005, 104,950 people will be diagnosed with colon cancer and 40,340 with rectal cancer. In the same year, an estimated 56,290 people will die of colorectal cancer. African Americans have a higher incidence of colorectal cancer then whites, and the mortality rate is also higher (21.1 percent among whites and 28.6 percent for African Americans. See Figure 6).

FIGURE 6

SEER Age Adjusted Incidence Rates by Race for Colon and Rectum
Cancer, All Ages, Both Sexes; SEER 9 Registries for 1973-2002; Age-
Adjusted to the 2000 US Std Population

Results:

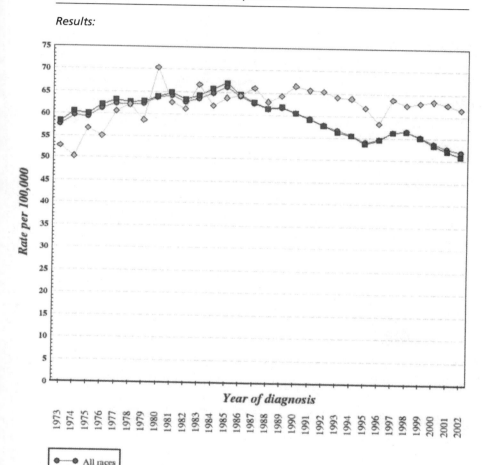

Year of diagnosis

All races
White
Black

Surveillance, Epidemiology, and End Results (SEER) Program (www.seer.cancer.gov) SEER*Stat
Database: Incidence - SEER 9 Regs Public-Use, Nov 2004 Sub (1973-2002), National Cancer Institute,
DCCPS, Surveillance Research Program, Cancer Statistics Branch, released April 2005, based on the
November 2004 submission.

As can be seen from Figure 6, the incidence has decreased over the years, although the decrease is less in African Americans.

PREVENTION OF COLORECTAL CANCER

Colorectal cancer is the fourth leading cause of cancer deaths in the United States; this may be due to the fact that it is often not diagnosed until the disease is in an advanced stage. For this reason, physicians are currently urging people of all races and ethnic groups to be screened regularly for any colon irregularities. In this way, patients with colorectal cancer can be treated early enough to stop the disease's progression.

Whether it is fear, embarrassment, or simply unfamiliarity of the disease, many people do not undergo necessary screening procedures (which will be discussed later in the chapter). Though colorectal cancer affects all ethnicities, African-Americans in particular are at a great risk, as they have the highest incidence of any minority. There is an increasing number of colon cancer outreach groups that are currently trying to educate the public about ways we all can help prevent the formation of cancer-causing agents.

In addition, proper diet, exercise, and screening by means of colonoscopy not only lessens the risk of colorectal cancer but can actually prevent it from occurring. While no single agent can prevent cancers, knowing how to eat properly can. By eating a variety of different foods, as described in Chapter 3, and maintaining a normal body weight, you greatly lower the odds that you might become a victim of this disease.

Preventing colorectal cancer isn't a one-shot. High-dose vitamins, minerals, or single dietary supplements have not proven to be effective in preventing cancers when tested in clinical trials. Ingesting a single pill or special elixir cannot make up for a risky lifestyle. Which leaves it with you: not to eat a healthy diet is high-risk behavior.

One important item of prevention diet is high fiber. In countries where a high fiber diet is the norm, the incidence of colorectal cancer is lower than in the United States. (Unfortunately, immigrants from these countries, once they have adapted to an American diet high in processed foods and low in fiber, will reach the same rates of colon cancer as the native United States population.

Diet alone doesn't work unless you also get proper exercise and control your weight. (Keep in mind that excess weight and obesity are risk factors in major killers like cancer, heart disease, and diabetes.) We African Americans are too ready to believe that we're just a naturally overweight people, and to take that as the norm. But we can change that norm. In fact, we *do* change it, one at a time, as we take our health in our own hands by eating right, keeping at a

FIGURE 7
ANATOMY OF THE COLON

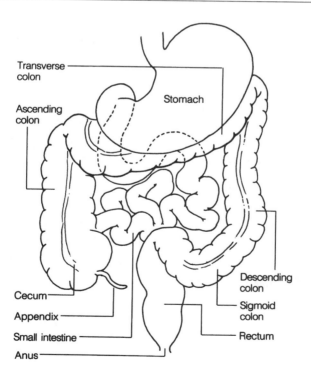

healthy weight, getting enough exercise, and avoiding things that are bad for the health, like smoking, drinking excessive alcohol, or taking street drugs.

THE TREATMENT TEAM

Once a patient has been diagnosed with colon cancer, there are many clinicians who will participate in the treatment of this disease. Because there are several different aspects to managing cancer, a collaborative approach requiring the skill and knowledge of different specialists is necessary. Some of the key members of the treatment team are:

Gastroenterologist: A gastroenterologist is a specialist in the diseases of the digestive tract ("gastro" means stomach, and "entero" relates to the intestines). A gastroenterologist will work closely with the other physicians on the team to ensure proper care. Frequently, it is the gastroenterologist who makes a diagnosis upon colonoscopy.

Surgeon: A surgeon will almost always intervene at some point in the care of a colorectal cancer patient. The surgeon is responsible for the resection, or removal, of any cancerous lesions along the digestive tract. He/she is usually a general surgeon who has some degree of expertise in these procedures.

ET Nurse: An Enterostomal Therapy (ET) nurse has received a specialized education in the care of patients who have any type of ostomy, like colostomy, resulting in an opening for waste removal. They are familiar with pre- and post-operative colorectal issues and the maintenance of a patient's colostomy.

Oncologist: An oncologist is a physician who manages patients with all types of cancer ("onco" means cancer, and "logy" means "the study of"). Your oncologist is the person who determines which chemotherapy medication will be the most effective. He/she works closely with your gastroenterologist as well as the other members of the treatment team.

SCREENING OF COLORECTAL CANCER

Colonoscopy is the best method we have for early detection of colorectal cancer. The procedure involves inserting a thin tube with an attached camera to visualize the entire inside surfaces of the colon and rectum. Doctors look for polyps and for the kind of cancer that arises from the inside lining of the colon. Because feces can obscure their visualization of the interior lining, it is necessary for you to flush all food out of the colon, before the colonoscopy. Your doctor will give you laxatives that take care of the flushing.

Laxatives are taken the day before the procedure. This process often proves more annoying then the actual procedure, which is generally done under light sedation. Laxatives can cause cramping and nausea, but while all that may make for an uncomfortable evening, most people get through it without serious complaint. Maybe it will help to think of it as an annual spring cleaning.

Although alternative means of screening for colorectal cancer exist, the colonoscopy remains the best method. Others include:

- Hemoccult tests that check for blood in a stool sample
- Sigmoidoscopy, which is a shorter version of the colonoscopy that inspects only the left side of the colon and not the entire colon
- Barium enema

But as a means of screening colon cancer these tests are a distant second to colonoscopy. They are still used and recommended as a screening method because they have been proven to be effective in large clinical trials, and they are widely available, and waiting times are shorter than for colonoscopy. They are cheaper, and less likely than colonoscopy to cause complications, though the complications are rare in any case.

If another screening method shows an abnormality, such as a polyp, no matter how small or seemingly insignificant, a colonoscopy needs to be done. My best advice is to have a colonoscopy when you reach fifty, and, if you're cancer free, you should have another one done ten years later. Healthy people at a high risk of developing colon cancer should have a repeat colonoscopy done every five years.

Some patients who are at a higher risk of colon cancer because they have had polyps in the past, have been placed on various vitamins and other agents in the hopes of preventing further development of colon cancer. A high fiber diet, vitamin C, and vitamin E have not proven effective in these high-risk groups. Other agents, such as selenium and calcium, have shown some benefit. Nonsteroidal anti-inflammatory drugs (NSAIDs) are the only agents that are in active use in preventing colon cancer.

Cancers of the colon develop from small growths called polyps, which are easily identified. There are two common types of polyps. One type, called hyperplasic polyps, rarely turn into cancer. The other type of polyp (adenomatous polyps) is more likely to turn into cancer.

The appearance of polyps is a signal that the person is at an increased risk of developing colon cancer in the future. If an adenomatous (or precancerous) polyp is found, a repeat colonoscopy is done within one to two years. If identified early, polyps can be removed during colonoscopy, and cancer will be prevented. A specialist called a gastroenterologist cuts out these small growths by using special attachments to the colonoscope.

It can take up to ten to fifteen years before a polyp will turn into a cancer. Given this long growth period, a colonoscopy only needs to be done every ten years, if the first test showed no polyps. If a polyp is seen and removed then a follow-up exam should be done to make sure that no other polyps have developed. Once a colon is free of polyps, a colonoscopy won't be needed for another ten years unless there is a family history of cancer.

New noninvasive technology is being introduced to do the job presently done by the colonoscopy. For example, a few centers are now screening for colon cancer by use of (a CT colonography) a CT scan that can examine the entire colon using x-ray. Although this procedure is in the early state of development and currently available at only a few sites, in the not-so-distant future, doctors are expected to make widespread use of virtual colonoscopy as a screening method.

TREATMENT OPTIONS

For cancers in the early stages, surgical removal offers an excellent chance of a cure. As mentioned above, certain polyps can be excised by polypectomy during a colonoscopy procedure. Some polyps in closer proximity to the anus may even be removed without the use of a scope by a procedure known as a transanal excision. Depending on the location of malignancy in the colon, it may be appropriate to remove only a segment; this is referred to as a partial colectomy. Under certain circumstances, it is necessary to remove the entire colon either to prevent or treat a cancerous spread.

In some of the cancers that exist near the sphincter, or the muscle that allows one to pass feces, it may be possible to maintain the musculature so that continence is preserved. However, because the sphincter itself may be cancerous, it is often necessary to include the sphincter in the surgical resection. In this case, the surgeon will create a colostomy through which feces may be excreted into an external bag.

If an organ such as the liver contains a solitary metastasic colorectal cancer lesion and there is no other evidence of distant metastatic disease, a patient such as this may benefit from a surgical resection of this solitary lesion.

Chemotherapy medications used in the treatment of colorectal cancer include oxaliplatin (Eloxatin), bevacizumab (Avastin), capecitabine (Xeloda), 5 fluorouracil (5-Fu), irinotecan (Camptosar) and cetuximab (Erbitux). Though these medicines are commonly used for metastatic disease and as adjuvant therapy, surgery remains the mainstay for the treatment of colon cancer.

In patients with colorectal cancer, either 5-FU or Xeloda will most likely be the prescribed course of treatment. There are very few chemical differences in these drugs; in fact, Xeloda is actually converted to 5-FU in the body before it begins combating cancer cells. Xeloda, as opposed to 5-FU, however, is taken orally, whereas 5-FU is given by IV (intravenously, or "into the veins"). If it is given by IV, it can be administered as either a bolus, or on "continuous infusion." The bolus injection usually takes under an hour to administer, whereas 5-FU given in continuous infusion can take up to 96 hours.

There are obvious advantages to taking Xeloda rather than 5-FU intravenously: being able to take a chemotherapy drug in the comfort of one's own home is certainly better than sitting in a hospital or a doctor's office for many hours. A patient receiving any intravenous drug might also encounter pain and discomfort associated with infections or irritations from the IV's incision. There are also various other complications that are possible from an IV drug, such as thrombosis (blood clots) or necrotic tissue (dead tissue) in the area surrounding the incision. However, because 5-FU is absorbed directly into the bloodstream, some patients might require this more direct injection of the drug depending on the stage and the type of cancer cells they demonstrate.

Surgery remains the mainstay for the treatment of colon cancer. Removing the cancer is the goal. For cancers in the early stages, surgical removal of small cancers offers excellent chances of cure.

Some of us are frightened by the word "surgery." But just as new technology is making screening exams far less uncomfortable for the patient, advances in surgery are similarly making surgery more patient friendly.

One new surgical technique allows surgeons to make only tiny incisions. A group of well-trained surgeons has learned to guide these small surgical instruments by use of video visualization, making the surgery far easier on the patient. Such techniques have been the standard in the removal of gallbladders, appendix, kidneys, and other organs, and it shouldn't be long before they're available to you.

Chemotherapy is a very powerful course of treatment, in that it attempts to destroy many cancer cells that are dividing uncontrollably. However, many of the body's healthy white cells, red cells, and platelets are affected in the process. The body's white cells, which are responsible for combating infection, are generally diminished in chemotherapy; this decrease in the body's immune defenses leads to infection, a primary side effect of chemotherapy. Other side effects include anemia, as a result of the chemotherapy destroying red blood cells, which also leads to fatigue. When the platelet levels are also reduced, the body's ability to stave off any bleeding is also weakened. This tendency to bleed is called thrombocytopenia, which is a common side effect of many chemo drugs.

Pain, hair loss, nausea, vomiting, and diarrhea are all additional side effects which should be discussed with your doctor. There are many remedies which may be able to help you through these difficult changes your body is experiencing. You may experience depression, anxiety, and fear during chemotherapy, and these emotions are entirely natural. It is important that you discuss your feelings either with friends and family members, or even support groups that are generally available through your hospital. Knowing that you are not alone may help ease the stress of your chemotherapy regimen.

COLOSTOMY

One result of surgery may be a colostomy. A colostomy is essentially an opening from the colon to the exterior of the abdomen. This colostomy acts as an anus through which the intestines may pass waste. Prior to the procedure, you may be asked to take enemas to ensure that the bowel is empty. Your physician might also prescribe antibiotics prior to surgery to minimize the risk of postoperative infection. After surgery, you may experience some pain upon breathing and sudden movement, but once the body begins to heal, normal activities may be resumed. Most patients who are to undergo a colostomy can expect few complications, though some risks may include wound infection, pneumonia, and pulmonary embolism.

An enterostomal therapy (ET) nurse will be of great assistance post-operatively. He/she will be able to advise you on how to care for your colostomy and help you get a pouch that is cut to fit your specific stoma size. There are many choices among ostomy supplies, and educating yourself on the many options will help you decide what is best for you. Generally, most pouches need to emptied every four to seven days. Initially, your ET nurse can help teach you how to empty and reattach your colostomy pouch. After your body has had time to heal and you've become accustomed to the care of your colostomy, you'll likely be able to maintain all of your regular activities and exercise, including swimming and bathing. Depending on the course of your illness after surgery, a colostomy may not interfere with even the most active lifestyle. Many patients become concerned with how a colostomy will affect their social and sexual life, but these activities do not need to change. Discussing your feelings with your close friends and romantic partners can only help you feel more comfortable with your life changes.

While colon cancer is a "common" cancer, it can be treated with excellent outcomes if caught early. Get a colonoscopy and see your doctor regularly. Prevention is the best way to reduce the odds on colon cancer.

IN A NUTSHELL

Incidence:
- Colon and rectal cancer, often referred to as "colorectal," are the third most common cancers in males and the second in females.
- In 2005, an estimated 104,950 people will be diagnosed with colon cancer and 40,340 with rectal cancer.

- In the same year, an estimated 56,290 people will die of colorectal cancer.
- African Americans have a higher incidence of colorectal then whites.

Cause:
Specific causes are thought to include:
- Genetic makeup
- Diet (cooking meat at high temperatures creates chemicals that cause cancer).

Prevention:
Eat a high-fiber diet containing fruits, grains, and vegetables.

Diagnosis:
- Be alert to any change in bowel habits or to blood in the stool.
- After age forty, ask your doctor for a digital rectal exam, a stool blood test, and a lower-colon exam (flexible sigmoidoscopy). You should get these tests every three to five years; they are covered by most health insurance policies.
- After age fifty, ask your doctor for a colonoscopy at the time of your regular colon checkup. It, too, is covered by most policies.

Treatment:
Surgery, in combination with chemotherapy when indicated.

Survival Rates:
Survival rates diminish dramatically according to the stage of the disease when diagnosed, but for each stage, African Americans are more likely to die than whites.

SEVEN

Lung Cancer

FROM HIS DOCTOR'S STANDPOINT, Frank's serious medical history began with a call from Frank's wife. Dr. Greenly had known Frank for ten years, since he'd come in with a variety of lung and breathing problems. The doctor would treat him, sometimes with antibiotics, sometimes with asthma inhalators. Each time, the doctor told Frank that the only meaningful prescription was to stop smoking. If smoking didn't ruin his heart, it would give him cancer in his lungs or somewhere else, the doctor would tell him. But Frank wasn't about to give up his habit. He'd been smoking his two packs a day for fifteen years, and he wasn't much over thirty. Worse still, because he didn't want to hear what Dr. Greenly had to tell him, he hadn't appeared for a routine exam, or for anything else, in more than two years.

So when Mary called to say that Frank was coughing constantly and losing weight, Dr. Greenly told her to bring him in right away. "Just ask the receptionist to make room for him this afternoon," he said.

Frank didn't come in that day or the next or the next. Dr. Greenly talked to Mary during that time, and she said Frank was just too afraid of cancer. But early the following week, Frank did come in, with Mary and his best friend, Thomas. It was Thomas who had finally persuaded Frank. By that time Frank's sputum was streaked with blood, so even he knew that he couldn't put the visit off any longer.

As soon as Frank walked into the examination room and took off his shirt, Dr. Greenly saw that he'd lost a lot of weight. He looked terrible, and the doctor knew that he must feel terrible. When Dr. Greenly heard a wheeze on the right side of Frank's chest, he knew that there was partial blockage of his right lung. Before Frank left the examination room, Dr. Greenly held the x-ray in his hand. There was a tumor in Frank's right lung.

> *Lung cancer is the number one cause of cancer deaths in the United States.*

Frank is typical when it comes to lung cancer. As more and more men smoked after both world wars, the incidence of cancer also increased. As more and more women took up the habit, the incidence of lung cancer among women increased as well.

That's why, though the disease was scarcely known of at the beginning of the twentieth century, in 2004, there was an estimated 173,770 new cases of lung cancer and it claimed an estimate of 160,440 lives. lung cancer today claims 170,000 or more new cases each year, and 150,000 lives. It is the number-one cause of cancer deaths in the United States.

Yet lung cancer isn't one of those diseases that we have little control over. If even half the African American smokers were to stop smoking tomorrow, and if we could teach our young people not to start, the rates of lung cancer would fall like a rock.

RISK FACTORS FOR LUNG CANCER

The percentage of Americans who smoke is declining each year, but, in 1997, about 6.7 million, or 14 percent of African-Americans still smoked. Between 1997 and 2001, African-American men had a

FIGURE 8

SEER INCIDENCE AND U.S. DEATH RATES, 1975–2002[†]

Lung and Bronchus Cancer, Both Sexes

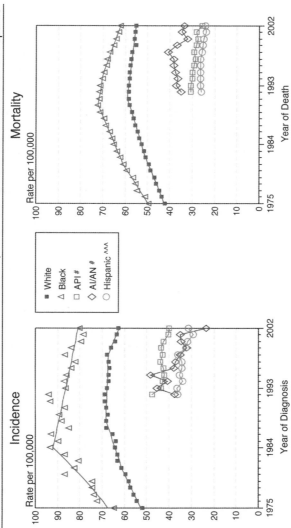

Joinpoint Analyses for 1975–2002 for Whites and Blacks
Rates for 1992–2002 for Asian/Pacific Islander, American Indian/Alaska Native and Hispanic

+ Source: Incidence data for whites and blacks is from the SEER 9 areas (San Francisco, Connecticut, Detroit, Hawaii, Iowa, New Mexico, Seattle, Utah, Atlanta). Incidence data for Asian/Pacific Islanders, American Indian/Alaska Natives and Hispanics is from the SEER 13 Areas (SEER 9 Areas, San Jose-Monterey, Los Angeles, Alaska Native Registry and Rural Georgia). Mortality data is from NCHS public use data file for the total US. Rates are age-adjusted to the 2000 US Std Population (19 age groups - Census P25-1103).
   Regression lines for whites and blacks are calculated using the Joinpoint Regression Program Version 3.0, April 2005, National Cancer Institute.
API = Asian/Pacific Islander. AI/AN = American Indian/Alaska Native.
^^^ Hispanic is not mutually exclusive from Whites, Blacks, Asian/Pacific Islanders, and American Indians/Alaska Natives. Incidence data for Hispanics excludes cases from Detroit, Hawaii, Alaska Native Registry and Rural Georgia. Mortality data for Hispanics excludes cases from Connecticut, Maine, Maryland, Minnesota, Oklahoma, New Hampshire, New York, North Dakota, and Vermont.

Surveillance, Epidemiology, and End Results (SEER) Program (www.seer.cancer.gov) SEER*Stat Database: Incidence - SEER 9 Regs Public-Use, Nov 2004 Sub (1973-2002), National Cancer Institute, DCCPS, Surveillance Research Program, Cancer Statistics Branch, released April 2005, based on the November 2004 submission.

death rate that was 36 percent higher than in white males. It kills more African Americans than any other cancer. African-American men are 50 percent more likely to develop long cancer than white men. These numbers translate into many cases of lung cancer and to many deaths.

Asbestos is also a high-risk factor. It can be found in many older homes that use asbestos insulation, and, if your job exposes you to asbestos, you may bring asbestos fibers home from work. Keep in mind that if you are exposed to environmental pollutants, smoking makes it worse. An asbestos worker who doesn't smoke has a risk of about seven times the normal. If that worker also smokes, the risk goes up to more than fifty to ninety times the normal.

Asbestos is part of a larger problem of environmental pollution. While the greatest percentage of lung cancer cases are caused by smoking, breathing bad air raises the risk of getting lung cancer at about the same rate as secondhand smoking does. Radon itself, a radioactive gas common in the air and in many homes, is the second leading cause of lung cancer in the United States and is associated with 15,000 to 22,000 lung cancer deaths each year.

Tobacco is a strong cancer-causing agent, associated with a number of different cancers, including lung cancer and other chronic lung diseases, as well as cardiovascular diseases.

AFRICAN AMERICANS AND LUNG CANCER

The "Annual Report to the Nation on the Status of Cancer, 1975–2002," published in the Oct. 5, 2005 issue of the *Journal of the National Cancer Institute*, shows observed cancer death rates from all cancers combined dropped 1.1 percent per year from 1993 to 2002.

Death rates from all cancers combined declined 1.5 percent per year from 1993 to 2002 in men, compared to a 0.8 percent decline in women from 1992 to 2002. Death rates decreased among men for twelve of the top fifteen cancers in men, and nine of the top fifteen cancers in women. Lung cancer is the leading cause of cancer deaths in both men and women.

African-American men, against males of all races, have the highest incidence rate of lung cancers, with an incidence rate of 117 per thousand, double the rate of most other races.

ANATOMY AND FUNCTION OF THE LUNG

First, let's take a short lesson on how the lungs work. The purpose of the lungs is to breathe in "good" air (oxygen) and breathe out "bad" air (carbon dioxide). There are two sets of lungs—right and left. Each is so efficient that a normal lung can do all the work alone if the other is removed. Each set is divided into segments, or lobes. There are three lobes on the right lung and two on the left. Each lobe

FIGURE 9
ANATOMY OF THE LUNGS

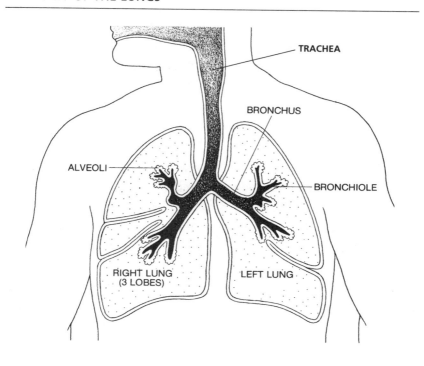

has multiple sacs or alveoli where oxygen and carbon dioxide are exchanged. These *alveoli* are connected by small tubes called *bronchioles* to larger tubes called *bronchi*. The bronchi, in turn, connect to a larger, central tube, the *trachea*, where air enters and leaves by way of the nose and the voice box or larynx.

The entire lung structure is lined with cells. These cells do the work of air exchange in the alveoli and clear the larger tubes (bronchioles and bronchi) of secretions. Any irritant, like tobacco smoke or certain environmental irritants, can cause changes in the cells and damage them. These changes can lead to cancer formation.

CAUSES OF LUNG CANCER

Before we return to lung cancer itself, we want to talk to you about its causes and prevention.

Although smoking is the major cause, there are other causes as well:

Environmental Pollution
While the greatest percentage of lung cancer cases are caused by smoking, breathing polluted air also raises the risk of getting lung cancer. As mentioned previously, radon, a radioactive gas common in the air and in many homes, is also a risk factor as is asbestos, and is associated with 15,000 to 22,000 lung cancer deaths each year.

Genetic Causes
Researchers have recently isolated three kinds of genes that may be involved. They are called *oncogenes*, which simply means genes related to oncology, or tumor-causing genes. One of these gene types is harmful to us, one is helpful, and the third, from all we know at this point, can act in either direction.

The first are proto-oncogenes, and they help to form tumors. The second are suppressor genes, and they obstruct tumor formation. The third are genes that produce enzymes to activate or inactivate carcinogens, which are substances that cause tumor formation.

HOW TOBACCO CAUSES CANCER

Though genetic and environmental perspectives are important, I don't want to obscure the core fact: the leading cause of lung cancer is tobacco.

It works like this. Smoke can directly damage the cells that line the tubes of the lung. It can also cause mutations in the genes that protect the lung from developing cancer.

The best way to stop lung cancer is to prevent it.

We've known since the U. S. Surgeon General's report in 1964 that cigarette smoking is the leading cause of cancer. Since then, evidence has given us a clearer and clearer picture:

- Risk of developing lung cancer increases in direct proportion to the number of cigarettes you smoke each day and the number of years you've been smoking.
- Smokers are estimated to run twenty times greater risk for lung cancer than nonsmokers. (They are also at twice the risk for stroke, six times for mouth cancer, ten times for larynx cancer, ten times for chronic obstructive pulmonary disease.)

The best way to stop lung cancer is to prevent it. Since 80 percent of lung cancers are attributed to smoking, it is obvious that many lives would be saved if people stopped smoking.

Thus our best prevention measures include the following:

- If you do smoke, stop smoking.
- If you don't smoke, don't start.
- Teach your children why their lives may depend on their not smoking.

From both a medical and economic viewpoint, it is astonishing that tobacco hasn't been outlawed. We worry a lot about drug and alcohol abuse, as we should, but tobacco addiction causes many more deaths.

Most of us know—even if some don't act on what they know—that tobacco is dangerous in all its forms. Pipe smoking, cigar smoking, snuff, chewed tobacco—all can kill you. African Americans are especially inclined to smoke mentholated cigarettes, probably because a tobacco company launched an effective advertising campaign to sell such cigarettes to us. The fact is that mentholated cigarettes can be particularly dangerous since the menthol encourages smokers to inhale more deeply and hold the smoke longer.

Remember, too, that it isn't the tobacco alone that can kill you. Tobacco smoke contains, besides nicotine, tar and other alkaloids and chemicals, some of them toxic. You might think twice if somebody invited you to smoke polycyclic hydrocarbons, benzopyrene, nitrosomines, and formaldehyde. But the fact is that you smoke all these every time you take a drag on a cigarette.

Tobacco is an addiction that hurts not only the smoker but the nonsmoker as well. In addition to the nearly half million preventable deaths it causes each year, it imposes an economic burden on nonsmokers, who must pay higher insurance premiums because of the high cost of tobacco-related illness, and who must also help pay for the medical treatment required by smokers without insurance.

If you, as a nonsmoker, live in a house with someone who smokes, your exposure to secondary smoke may be dangerous to your health.

If you, as a nonsmoker, live in a house with someone who smokes, your exposure to secondary smoke may be dangerous to your health. If you raise a child in a household where others smoke, the child, too, may suffer from damaged lungs.

Finally, remember that tobacco can be harmful not only to your lungs but to your heart as well. Your risk of heart failure and coronary artery disease is much greater if you smoke. So, incidentally, is your risk of gum disease and eventual tooth loss.

We think that every smoker owes it to himself or herself to stop. They owe it also to their loved ones, whom they place at risk. They owe it to those who depend on them not to risk their lives so recklessly. But above all, they owe it to their children.

Tobacco companies have been especially successful in targeting our children. In 2004, a total of 11.7 percent of middle school students reported current use of a tobacco product. While such rates are dropping, they still show that far too many of our young people are putting themselves at risk for lung cancer and for other types of cancer as well.

If you yourself are a smoker, the best way to discourage your children from taking up the habit is through your own good example. Stop smoking. Although some of the damage you've already done to your lungs may prove permanent, other functions of the lung will heal. Your lungs will recover their ability to remove mucus. Your risk of cancer will diminish, and if you stay clean for fifteen to twenty years, that risk won't be much higher than that of people who never smoked. Your risk of getting emphysema will be reduced as much as six times. Finally, your risk of heart disease is halved in the first year, and in about five years approaches that of nonsmokers.

Kicking the habit will help you in other, less dramatic ways as well. Your breath and clothes will no longer reek of tobacco, and your fingers and nails will no longer be stained with it. The sores you may have developed in your mouth as a result of smoking will heal and vanish. You'll miss fewer days from work (and from play) because of sickness. You will enjoy the sheer body energy of being healthy, and that will give you greater pleasure in many activities. You'll even enjoy your food more.

Yes, increased appetite can raise a problem. People can gain weight after they stop smoking. But you can learn to satisfy the new appetite by snacking on fruits and vegetables. They're good in themselves, and they won't add to your weight. Besides, they'll help take your mind off high-calorie snacks. In any case, average weight gains are small (5 to 10 pounds) for people who do gain weight.

Many people start exercising when they stop smoking. It keeps their weight down, is good for the heart, and helps let their body know that they are really serious about treating it kindly. You may find that your self-image as a healthy, vigorous person becomes a kind of addiction itself, especially when others tell you how good you're looking.

HOW TO STOP SMOKING

Here's what has worked for others and can work for you:

1. Set a date and time for quitting and stick to it.
2. Picture yourself as a person who has successfully stopped smoking.
3. Chew gum, eat plenty of fruits and vegetables, and absolutely avoid coffee and alcohol. You know how comfortably cigarettes go with coffee and alcohol.
4. Don't let your body dwell on cigarettes. Keep your hands busy. And give your body another focus: play sports, exercise, or take frequent cold showers or baths.
5. While you're working on this big change, buy some new clothes, get your teeth cleaned, maybe even change your hairstyle. The fact is you've chosen to start your life over, and, like a good actor, you need a few props or costume changes to help you with this new character.
6. Read all you can about the effects of smoking and about people who have quit. Maybe find a friend who also wants to quit. You can help each other out. And avoid friends who do smoke, or politely ask them not to smoke around you. If they're truly your friends, they'll be glad to oblige.
7. If you are religious and believe in the Lord, ask your minister and fellow church members to pray for you, and ask the Lord for help in this endeavor.

8. Reward yourself each day that you don't smoke. Not with fattening food, please. You already know about that. But give yourself a treat that's good for your body or your soul. You might give yourself a bigger reward for each week or month that you've kept yourself clean of nicotine.
9. When possible, avoid the smoking sections of restaurants and airports.
10. Keep notes in your pocket or on a little laminated card stating that you've quit and the reasons why.
11. Listening to music, reading a book, and working at a hobby are all ways of resisting the urge to smoke.
12. Keep telling yourself you can quit. You can. You will.

Remember: many Americans stop smoking every year. What they have done you can do.

SYMPTOMS AND DETECTION OF LUNG CANCER

A new cough, or a change in the quality of a cough, is often what brings the patient in for a lung examination. Lung cancer is also sometimes detected on a routine chest x-ray, which discloses a "coin" lesion, a small, round tumor. At its earliest stage of development, that tumor will not cause symptoms. If it is allowed to grow, however, it will irritate the bronchial tubes (small airway passages in the lung) and cause a cough.

When a patient comes in complaining about a chronic cough, especially if the patient is a smoker, the doctor will want to find the specific cause. If the tumor has developed far enough to ulcerate, some blood may be visible when coughing. The bleeding is rarely massive.

If the tumor has begun to block the bronchial tube, the patient will experience shortness of breath, and the doctor will detect wheezing on one side. (The patient may also experience chest pain if the tumor has invaded the nerves in that area.) If the tumor *completely* blocks the part of our breathing apparatus called the *bronchus*, lung secretions will get trapped there and make breathing difficult, or even cause infection. (The tumor may form a cavity in the lung, and, without the help of a biopsy, that may be mistaken for tuberculosis.) Pneumonia may be an early warning.

In lung cancer as in all cancers, *early diagnosis offers the best chance of recovery and cure.* The longer a lung tumor is allowed to grow, the more trouble it will cause. Tumors in the upper part of the lung (apex) can invade ribs or nerves, causing pain or even local paralysis of muscle—in the arm or hand, for instance.

> *Early diagnosis offers the best chance of recovery and cure.*

If the tumor continues to enlarge, it may also block important blood vessels, causing swelling of the face or arms. Often a lung tumor grows into the central chest area, invading the nerve to the voice box and causing hoarseness. When that happens, surgical removal of the tumor is no longer possible.

Metastases from lung cancers are common, especially to the brain, liver, and bone.

Sometimes the cancer itself produces abnormal hormones, which can result in an odd set of symptoms that might seem to have little to do with the lung: skin rash, arthritis, muscular weakness, bleeding and coagulation problems, anemia, or urinary abnormalities are all possible.

See your doctor immediately if you have the following set of symptoms:

- Cough
- Blood-streaked sputum.
- Loss of appetite
- Weight loss.

DIAGNOSIS

Doctors have several methods available to diagnose lung cancer:

- A "presumptive" diagnosis can be made from the sputum, examined under a microscope by a pathologist.
- An x-ray of the lung will reveal any lesion, whether it is a cancer or not.
- Newer scanning devices, like CT (a computerized x-ray procedure) or MRI (magnetic resonance imaging) reveal more detail than the routine x-ray. These newer devices provide more information about how deeply the tumor is attached to the lung and whether the disease has spread.
- The doctor can directly observe tumors located in the bronchi with the use of a device called a *bronchoscope*. With this device, the doctor can biopsy the tumor and, by determining its exact location, decide whether the tumor can be removed. (If the tumor is peripheral—that is, close to the chest wall—a biopsy can also be obtained by means of a needle inserted through the chest wall.)
- Another device, called a *thoroscope*, can also be used if the tumor is peripheral. Thoroscopy also allows the doctor to view the lining of the chest cavity for other possible tumor implants. It is inserted directly into the chest, the patient having been anesthetized.
- Finally, the central part of the chest (mediastinum) can be evaluated for possible spread of tumor to this area by making a small neck incision and inserting a lighted instrument called a *mediastinoscope*. Such an evaluation is commonly used in the process of staging.

Obviously, doctors go to great lengths in obtaining a good specimen (piece of tumor). That's because treatment depends on the specific type of tumor. The common types are:

- The small cell lung cancer (SCLC), formally called *oat cell cancer* because the cells are small like grains of oats

- Nonsmall cell lung cancer (NSCLC)

SCLC makes up about 20 percent of cancer cells, and NSCL about 75 percent. The other 5 percent are rare: lymphoma, metastatic melanoma, carcinoids, and so forth.

Even though all these tests are useful, in the case of lung cancer, as of all cancers, the final diagnosis depends on biopsy.

STAGING LUNG CANCER

As in all cancers, staging lung cancer is essential. Only through staging can we determine the kind and extent of treatment. Only through staging can your doctor say, with any degree of accuracy, your chance of cure or your life expectancy. Here is one of the standard staging systems for lung cancer. As you will see from it, stages I and II have a fair prognosis, but stages III and IV are, with few exceptions, hopeless.

MANAGING LUNG CANCER

The management of lung cancer depends on the stage of the cancer and the overall health of the patient. The treatment for lung cancer may involve surgery, radiation, and/or chemotherapy. If the lung cancer is at an early stage (IA–IIIA) and the patient's overall health is adequate to handle it, surgery is the first option. Patients who don't meet these criteria may be candidates for chemotherapy and/or radiation therapy.

When surgery reveals that the lymph nodes are involved in the cancer, chemotherapy after surgery is usually recommended to lessen the chance that the cancer will return. Patients viewed as poor surgical candidates, if the cancer is stage IIIB or less, may be candidates for a combined treatment of chemotherapy and radiation.

Patients who are found to have extensive lung cancer at the time of diagnosis or later may also be candidates for the new target

TABLE 3
STAGES OF LUNG CANCER

STAGE	DIAGNOSIS	PROGNOSIS
Stage 0	Carcinoma *in-situ* (the cancer hasn't yet invaded the basement membrane)	Good
Stage I	Tumor arising 2 cm or more from junction of right and left bronchi. No extension into lymph nodes. No involvement of lung covering	Fair
Stage II	Same as stage I, but lymph nodes in mediastinum (central chest) are involved	Fair to poor
Stage III	Extension of tumor to chest wall and nearby organs, like heart	Poor
Stage IV	Spread of tumor to distant organs (liver, bones, etc.)	Poor

therapies. Tarceva®, which is a tyrosine kinase inhibitor, has been found to be effective in lung cancer. Tyrosine kinases are enzymes that help certain cancer cells grow and spread. Unlike most chemotherapy medications, these agents are not IV medications, but are taken orally. Use of these medications should be considered in patients with advanced disease and who have already been given other treatments.

THE COURSE OF FRANK'S ILLNESS

When Frank appeared in Dr. Greenly's office with a more intense cough that produced blood-streaked sputum, the doctor ordered an x-ray. It revealed a large irregular mass in the right lung. A CT scan gave a clearer picture: the mass was in the lower portion of the right lung. There was evidence of lymph nodes present in the central chest (mediastinum).

Mediastinoscopy, obtained by inserting a tube, allowed a view of the mediastinum. The doctor made a short incision in Frank's neck and inserted the tube. A few lymph nodes were removed for microscopic examination.

The lymph nodes were negative. Other tests suggested that his general condition was strong enough to withstand a major chest operation. Frank did get through the operation with flying colors. (The final pathology showed this to be a 3-cm cancer—NSCLC.) Now, six months later, he's recovered well and—it goes without saying—he no longer smokes.

Emotionally, he's had to make some adjustments. It isn't always easy to live with the knowledge that his chances of surviving five years are 50 percent. But he's grown philosophical about it. What he said one night over dinner with Mary and their friends, Thomas and his wife Jasmine, was that he was beginning to enjoy living one day at a time. "You know," he said, "it gives my life an intensity it didn't have in the old days. Times like this, with the people I love, have a deeper sweetness. It's the same when I play with the kids. It's the same even at work. It's like I'm finally where I ought to have been from the beginning, tasting every moment for the last drop of deliciousness that's in it."

Frank's was a hard way to learn. But sometimes the hard way is the only way there is.

WHAT'S NEW IN LUNG CANCER?

A recent article in the *Journal of the National Cancer Institute* reports that women smokers are twice as likely to develop lung cancer than men. It turns out that a gene that causes abnormal growth of lung cells is more active in women. Female smokers who have that active gene are at 12 times higher risk than a nonsmoker, whereas male smokers who have it are at 2.4 times higher risk.

The lesson seems obvious. *Women have even a greater reason than men to stop smoking.*

Interesting work has also been done on the mineral selenium. In patients with lung cancer, the concentration of selenium in blood and lung tissue is decreased. That decrease is associated with a decrease in antioxidant activity and with the progression of the disease. This suggests that selenium as a food supplement is probably a good idea in lung cancer patients.

For healthy people, too, supplementary selenium may make sense. Selenium appears to discourage the growth of blood vessels that cancer cells need to grow and spread.

We also know that special care must be taken to protect lung cancer patients from diseases like pneumonia and other infections. Lung cancer patients suffer weakening of their immune systems and are especially vulnerable to such infection. They and the people who care for them should wear face masks and wash their hands frequently. A diet heavy in fruits and vegetables is especially important because such a diet helps strengthen the immune system.

Finally, exciting work is going on in several hospitals. Memorial Sloan-Kettering Cancer Center has made intraoperative (that is, in the operating room while the chest is open) irradiation part of their treatment of lung cancer. They find that there is improved survival but no added complications. Mt. Vernon Hospital in the United Kingdom has increased the frequency of x-ray treatment to every eight hours to decrease the proliferation of cancer cells between the ordinary courses of x-ray therapy. Survival rates of their patients have improved modestly.

IN A NUTSHELL

Incidence:
- African-American men have the highest incidence of lung cancers.
- African-American women have the highest incidence of lung cancers.
- Lung cancer is epidemic among African-American males.

Cause:
Smoking is the main cause for lung cancer.

Prevention:
- Lung cancer is the most preventable of all cancers.
- Stop smoking.
- Avoid asbestos and radon.

Diagnosis:
- Get a lung x-ray once a year.
- Be alert to such symptoms as a steady cough, blood-streaked sputum, and loss of appetite, especially if these symptoms accompany cigarette smoking.

Treatment:
Lung cancer is treated by chemotherapy plus x-ray treatment, and/or, in worst cases, removal of part of the lung.

Prognosis:
Prognosis for lung cancer is fair for stage I, poor for stage II, and still poorer for stages III and IV.

EIGHT

Cancer of the Prostate

MY FRIEND NATHAN CALLED ME one night several years back to tell me he was scheduled for surgery the next day. We chatted for a while, and I reassured him as well as I could. Nathan had gone in for a physical exam recently, after a five-year lapse. "Why do I need to see a doctor?" he'd say to his wife, "I'm feeling fine."

But his doctor had diagnosed a nodule on his prostate, and, when the pathology results came in, the diagnosis was cancer. The operation he faced that morning was a radical prostatectomy—that is, removal of the prostate gland.

Nathan knew the operation would mean pain and discomfort, and could have long-term effects on his sexual functioning. Nathan was a strong man who, at sixty-eight, had learned more than once how to draw on the strength he needed to get through bad times. But like most men, Nathan felt deeply threatened by the prospect of lifelong impotence, and I gave him what comfort I could.

I visited him after surgery. The operation had gone perfectly and he seemed in as good spirits as a man can be after such an ordeal.

The pathology reports brought good news as well: there was no lymph node involvement. That meant, of course, that there were no signs of metastasis.

But before long, serious problems began to set in. Nathan had trouble getting an erection, and though his wife couldn't have been more understanding, Nathan's sense of himself as a man was threatened.

As bad as this was, worse still perhaps is that he was incontinent, that is, unable to control his urine. It pained him deeply to find himself wearing what he insisted on calling "diapers." What's more, he developed swelling in both legs. That, at least, his doctor could treat—with blood thinners and leg stockings, but Nathan considered the stockings themselves just one more humiliation. Nathan was a strong man, but his spirit had been brought low by his disease.

Not only are African Americans more likely than whites to suffer from prostate cancer, but they are more likely to die from it.

One day about six months after the operation, I called Nathan's house and his wife answered. He was gone, she told me—just a week ago. An *embolism* (blood clot) got into the lungs and he died suddenly.

Nathan's story is typical, but it didn't have to happen that way. If he had been getting annual checkups, his cancer would have been detected earlier. If he had been eating a high-fiber diet, including fruits, grains, and vegetables, he might never have gotten cancer at all.

PROSTATE CANCER AND THE AFRICAN-AMERICAN MAN

Prostate cancer is a threat to men of all races, but it is particularly a threat to African Americans, who are more than twice as likely to die of it. By 2002, the rate of prostate cancer deaths was 26.2/100,000 men for whites, but for African Americans rate was 64.0/100,000 men.

FIGURE 10

SEER INCIDENCE AND U.S. DEATH RATES, 1975–2002[†]

Prostate Cancer

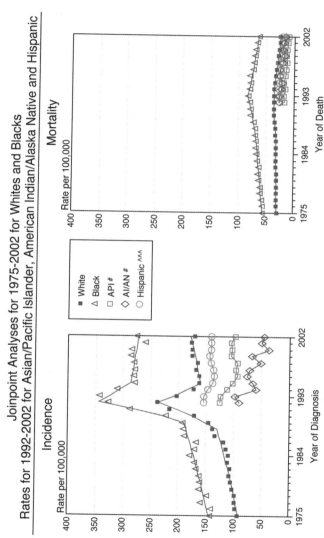

Joinpoint Analyses for 1975-2002 for Whites and Blacks
Rates for 1992-2002 for Asian/Pacific Islander, American Indian/Alaska Native and Hispanic

Incidence

Mortality

Year of Diagnosis

Year of Death

- White
- Black
- API #
- AI/AN #
- Hispanic ^^^

[†] Source: Incidence data for whites and blacks is from the SEER 9 areas (San Francisco, Connecticut, Detroit, Hawaii, Iowa, New Mexico, Seattle, Utah, Atlanta). Incidence data for Asian/Pacific Islanders, American Indian/Alaska Natives and Hispanics is from the SEER 13 Areas (SEER 9 Areas, San Jose-Monterey, Los Angeles, Alaska Native Registry and Rural Georgia). Mortality data is from NCHS public use data file for the total US. Rates are age-adjusted to the 2000 US Std Population (19 age groups - Census P25-1103). Regression lines for whites and blacks are calculated using the Joinpoint Regression Program Version 3.0, April 2005, National Cancer Institute.

\# API = Asian/Pacific Islander. AI/AN = American Indian/Alaska Native.

^^^ Hispanic is not mutually exclusive from Whites, Blacks, Asian/Pacific Islanders, and American Indians/Alaska Natives. Incidence data for Hispanics excludes cases from Detroit, Hawaii, Alaska Native Registry and Rural Georgia. Mortality data for Hispanics excludes cases from Connecticut, Maine, Maryland, Minnesota, Oklahoma, New Hampshire, New York, North Dakota, and Vermont.

Surveillance, Epidemiology, and End Results (SEER) Program (www.seer.cancer.gov) SEER*Stat Database: Incidence - SEER 9 Regs Public-Use, Nov 2004 Sub (1973-2002), National Cancer Institute, DCCPS, Surveillance Research Program, Cancer Statistics Branch, released April 2005, based on the November 2004 submission.

A key reason for this gap is that African-American and Hispanic men are likely to be diagnosed with prostate cancer later in the course of the disease than are white men. Men who are diagnosed early are men more likely to survive. To get the best chance of being successfully treated, diagnosis before the disease is a year old is optimal. Each year of delay decreases the odds of being successfully treated. We think it's important for the health and longevity of African-American men thirty to thirty-five years old and older to get a physical checkup once a year. If you already have a doctor, you are hopefully getting such checkups already. If you don't have one, and can't afford to pay for necessary treatments, go to the Web site for the Centers for Medicare and Medicaid Services, *www.cms.hhs.gov/*. There you will find information to help you get the best medical treatment possible, regardless of your income. One good support group is the Prostate Health Education Network (PHEN), affiliated with the Dana-Ferber Institute, *www.prostate-healthed.org/*. This group was formed to support African-American men facing this disease.

ANATOMY AND FUNCTION OF
THE PROSTATE

The prostate is a gland located below the bladder that surrounds the upper part of the tube leading from the bladder through the penis to the end of the penis. About the size of a walnut and shaped like a chestnut, the prostate produces a thick fluid that empties into the urethra and forms part of the semen. The function of the prostate is controlled by the hormone testosterone, which is produced primarily in the testicles.

CAUSES OF PROSTATE CANCER

The exact causes of this cancer, a malignant tumor in the prostate, are unknown. But we do know the formation of the tumor is related to

FIGURE 11
ANATOMY OF THE PROSTATE

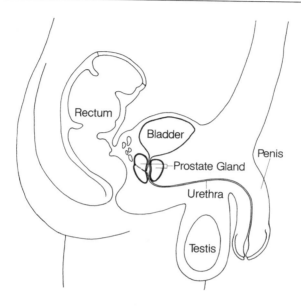

Rectum

Bladder

Penis

Prostate Gland

Urethra

Testis

the production of testosterone, which acts directly on the cells of the prostate. Some irregularity in the testosterone causes these cells to divide abnormally, and their excessive growth can result in a tumor.

Even within this irregular pattern, the development may take place in an orderly fashion and not spread to adjacent or distant organs. In such a case, the process is benign and is known as *benign prostatic hypertrophy*, or, in ordinary language, enlargement of the prostate gland. Although benign, this process can cause a backup of urine by obstructing the urethra. It will then require surgery.

When the cells become angry-looking and spread to other organs, the process becomes malignant.

Although we don't know enough yet to say what sets this process in motion, there are a number of risk factors:

- Diets high in fat are a risk factor. That is one of many reasons (the danger of heart disease, breast cancer, and diabetes are among others) why it's so important that we cut down as far as possible the amount of fat in our diet.

- Race
- Old age itself is a risk factor. In sixty-five-year-old men, the incidence of prostate cancer is 35 percent. For men age ninety, the rate more than doubles, to 75 percent. We should add, however, that a good number of these cases aren't severe enough as to require treatment.
- Strong family history of prostate cancer.

SYMPTOMS AND DIAGNOSIS

Over time, a tumor of the prostate progressively squeezes and blocks the urethra it surrounds, obstructing the passage of urine. The resulting symptoms are:

- Difficulty urinating
- Increased frequency of urinating
- Urgency of urinating
- Trouble completely emptying the bladder
- Possible dribbling.

Diagnosis of prostate cancer has improved greatly with the discovery of the tumor marker PSA.

Diagnosis of prostate cancer has improved greatly with the discovery of the tumor marker named *prostate-specific antigen* (PSA). Unfortunately, despite its name, it is *not* specific. A urinary infection and other irregularities can cause a rise in PSA. So can a condition called BPH (benign prostatic hypertrophy). But the accuracy of the test is improving.

After ordering the PSA test, which is a simple blood test, the doctor will perform a prostate rectal exam. (Determining the PSA *after* the rectal exam may yield a false-positive elevation.) If the doctor feels a mass in the prostate, he will order a needle biopsy.

Where the doctor doesn't feel a mass but the PSA is elevated, the patient may be put on antibiotics for several weeks. If the problem is infection of the prostate, the PSA should disappear under antibiotic treatment. But if the condition doesn't disappear, the doctor will order a *rectal ultrasound* (US). On the basis of what the US shows, biopsies of other suspicious areas may be needed. If the PSA remains high and no new areas are discovered through the US, a *blind biopsy* (biopsy of six randomly selected areas) may be performed.

Other tests usually ordered in the case of a sustained high PSA level are the *intravenous pyelogram* (IVP), which evaluates the kidney, and *cystoscopy*—which allows the doctor to look with a light through the penis into the bladder—in order to evaluate the bladder.

Where there is an obstruction, a *urologist*—a surgeon specializing in the urinary system—can sometimes correct it surgically.

TREATMENT

Treatment depends on what stage the cancer has reached. The stage system outlined here is based on the National Cancer Institute's pamphlet on prostate cancer (No. 96–175):

- Stage I: Tumor is not evident by rectal exam and is without specific symptoms.
- Stage II: Tumor is felt as nodule on rectal exam and confined to prostate.
- Stage III: Cancer has spread beyond prostate to nearby tissues.
- Stage IV: Cancer has spread to lymph nodes or other organs.

Because there are several options for treatment, it's a good idea to get a second opinion and then make your choice between the following treatments:

1. Observe without treatment. In the case of older men, particularly, many authorities recommend that careful monitoring is the best course.

2. Surgical removal of prostate and lymph nodes, with lymph node dissection for staging. Only patients in good medical condition are suitable for this surgery. Age is also a consideration.
3. Radiation therapy—suitable for stage II and sometimes stage III if the local spread isn't too extensive. At stage IV, radiation treatment may relieve pain.
4. Hormone treatment that either (a) blocks or eliminates testosterone by removing the testicles, or (b) introduces the female hormone *stilbestrol*. Metastatic lesions have been seen to be controlled or even "melt away" as a result of hormone therapy.
5. Other therapies more rarely employed in the treatment of prostate cancer are cryosurgery (freezing) and chemotherapy.

A NOTE ON RADIATION TREATMENT FOR PROSTATE CANCER

When one is diagnosed with *early-stage* prostate cancer, the discussion about treatment options can become confusing. Surgery, radiation, hormonal shots, alone or in combination, are all viable options. For men suffering from other life-threatening diseases such as heart or chronic pulmonary disease, simple observation with no active therapy for the prostate cancer may be the best choice available. Small, early-stage prostate cancer tends to grow slowly. Treating a prostate cancer in these instances may not prolong life and, just as important, will not improve the quality of life. Small prostate cancers that are only discovered on the basis of an increase in the PSA blood test do not cause symptoms.

It is helpful in these circumstances to seek a second or even third opinion. A urologist (a surgeon who specializes in diseases of the urinary system, which includes the prostate gland) will provide the best information concerning the risks and benefits of surgical resection—a *prostatectomy* (removing the prostate). Radiation therapy is best discussed with a radiation therapist.

Once it is decided that surgery is not the best option and that radiation therapy is the way to go, the specific method of radiation therapy becomes important. Yes, even in the area of radiation therapy there are choices to be made.

The different approaches used in radiation will have a lot to do with what is available in the community. Because this is a high-tech area of treatment, it is ever changing. A heavy reliance on computers and other high-tech devices means that not all facilities are capable of delivering all the available treatment modalities.

The most widely available type of radiation treatment, and the one most commonly used in treating early-stage disease, is external beam radiotherapy, more specifically called *conventional external beam radiotherapy. Conformal radiotherapy* and *brachytherapy* are the other two methods increasingly becoming available.

To understand the basic differences between these techniques as treatment of early-stage prostate cancer requires a simple explanation of the general risks and benefits of radiation.

Radiation therapy works by delivering a dose of powerful x-rays to the prostate gland containing the cancer. A higher dose of radiation results in more tissue being destroyed, and with it, the cancer. If a small portion of the cancer is located outside of the area or field of the x-rays, then it is spared, and remains capable of growing and spreading to other areas of the body (metastasis). It is therefore of utmost importance that all the cancer be included in the field of the x-rays. This is why only early-stage prostate cancer can be treated for cure with radiation.

In addition to destroying the prostate cancer, radiation will damage any tissue it penetrates in reaching the target. Because the prostate gland is situated deep in the pelvis surrounded by primarily the rectum and bladder, injury to these structures is possible if the x-ray beam is not carefully aimed. When such injury occurs, bowel, bladder, and sexual function commonly become problematic in the post-treatment period.

All of the newer current techniques in radiation therapy are geared to 1) limiting the area of radiation exposure to only the prostate gland and 2) achieving a higher dose of radiation to this target area. Conventional radiation targets a wider area of treatment including the prostate and a portion of the rectum and bladder. Conventional radiation cannot be given in high doses because the rectum and bladder would be severely injured. It is used in those cases where the cancer may have spread beyond the prostate gland.

Conformal radiotherapy is a technique that specifically targets only the prostate gland. Special CT scans of the prostate gland are taken so that a true three-dimensional map can be made of the gland. Computers are used to define as accurately as possible the entire surface of the prostate gland. The x-ray beam is then fashioned with special blocks so that the x-ray beam matches or conforms to the exact shape of the prostate gland. The surrounding structures are thus avoided. A higher dose of radiation can then be given, resulting in greater destruction of the cancer. To make sure that the patient does not move during the x-ray treatment and that the same position is used over the course of treatment, a custom-made mold is used to stabilize the patient during treatment. The patient is immobilized in the exact same position each time. This assures that no normal structures get in the way.

In order to achieve a curative dose of radiation, multiple treatments are required. A large dose cannot be given all at once. The patient frequently must undergo treatments Monday through Friday and for five to six weeks.

Another technique, called *brachytherapy,* can sometimes be used as treatment. Here, the actual source of radiation, in the form of small radioactive seeds, is permanently implanted into the prostate gland. These seeds are so small that they are placed through a small needle inserted into the prostate gland at the time of surgery.

Advantages of this approach include the following:

- It is a one-time application of radiation. Patients don't have to receive repeated daily treatments as in the case of external beam.
- It is an outpatient procedure, and no major surgical procedure is required.
- It involves little risk to surrounding areas because the seeds are placed within the gland.
- It requires no major change in the quality of life after treatment. The patient can be back to work in a few days.

Again, only early-stage patients are candidates for brachytherapy. Further, the technique is just becoming more readily available in the community setting. Complications, when they occur, can be significant. A combination of external radiation and brachytherapy may prove beneficial in patients with more advanced disease.

As treatment options continue to expand, patient education becomes more important so they understand the risks and benefits of each approach. In early-stage prostate cancer there is time for the patient and physician to make final treatment decisions carefully and without haste. Participating in clinical trials often assures that the best approach will be used, and it also allows the patient to know that his treatment may make possible better treatment options for other patients.

COMPLICATIONS THAT MAY FOLLOW TREATMENT

Surgery, as we've said, may result in erectile dysfunction and incontinence. Recent innovations, by sparing nerves, allow an erection. In addition, the surgeon now spares a longer segment of the urethra, and that helps save the patient from the annoyance of incontinence.

Swelling of the legs (*phlebitis* or clots in the veins) can also be a serious problem, and the result can be life-threatening *pulmonary emboli* (clots to the lung), as it was in Nathan's case.

Because each of the possible therapies for prostate cancer carries risks of its own, it's especially important that the patient ask questions, seek a second opinion, and, if he decides on a prostatectomy, be certain that the urologist he chooses has successfully performed a number of these operations. Whatever therapy you choose, ask questions.

QUESTIONS TO ASK IF YOU CHOOSE SURGERY

- Can I just wait?
- What are my chances of cure with the operation?
- How long will it take me to fully recover?
- How does the benefit and risk of surgery compare with that of x-ray therapy?
- Will the surgery affect my sex life?
- Will I have trouble urinating and controlling urine?
- Are there clinical trials, and what are the advantages of my entering one?

QUESTIONS TO ASK IF YOU CHOOSE RADIATION THERAPY

- How do the benefits and risks of radiation compare with those of surgery?
- Will the treatments affect my sex life?
- How many treatments will I need?
- Can I continue working during treatment? If not, how soon after?
- Will the treatments be painful?

QUESTIONS TO ASK IF YOU CHOOSE HORMONAL THERAPY

- Will it control the disease?
- How do its benefits and risks compare with those of surgery and radiation?
- Will my voice change, or will I experience other changes as a result of the female hormone?
- Will I still be able to have an erection after treatment?

IN A NUTSHELL

Incidence:

Among males, cancer of the prostate is the most common cancer; it is still more common among African Americans and has a higher death rate. For the year 2000, the American Cancer Society estimates 180,100 new cases of prostate cancer, with an estimated 31,000 deaths. In 2000–2003 the incidence of prostate cancer in African Americans is 258.3 per 100,000; for whites, 163.4 per 100,000.

Cause:

The cause of prostate cancer is unknown, but suspected causes include fatty diet, vasectomy, employment in rubber factories, and age itself.

Prevention:

Besides diet, the best protection is regular PSA and rectal exams after the age of fifty.

Diagnosis:

- Be alert to frequent need to urinate and dribbling, or of blood in your urine.
- Every man over the age of forty should have a digital rectal examination as part of his regular annual physical checkup.

- After the age of fifty, all men should have an annual PSA blood test. If the results of either test are suspicious, a technique known as transrectal ultrasound can be used to reveal cancers too small to be detected through a physical exam.

Treatment:
Observation (where PSA levels are relatively low), radical prostatectomy, x-ray, hormonal therapy, cryosurgery (rare).

Prognosis:
Good (75 percent) if diagnosed and treated early. For patients who have had radical prostatectomy and radiation therapy, five-year survival rates are 75 percent, ten-year survival rates 60 percent. Fewer than 10 percent of such patients suffer incontinence.

Potency after a radical prostatectomy varies according to age:
50 percent in a fifty-year-old man, 20 percent at age seventy.

Possible complications from treatment:
Erectile dysfunction; incontinence; blood clots in legs.

NINE

Thyroid Cancer

M Y OWN STRUGGLE WITH CANCER began more than twenty years ago. I was shaving on a bright spring morning when I first noticed a swelling on my neck the size of a golf ball. When I swallowed, it moved up and down. I knew at once what it was. I'd felt a hundred such thyroid nodules in my own patients.

I also knew the percentages—and you can be sure that I was weighing them at that moment. Only 5 percent of single thyroid nodules are malignant, I reminded myself. Pretty good odds. But survival depends on the type of the tumor, and I wouldn't know that until I'd had tests.

My surgeon ordered the then usual thyroid tests:

- Scan
- Ultrasound
- Thyroid function tests.

If I'd been diagnosed today, I also would have had a needle biopsy.

The first test results were very hopeful: a benign adenoma—that is, a noncancerous tumor in the gland, just as my mother had ten years earlier. But when they examined the tumor after removing it, the story took a different turn. *Follicular cancer,* the pathology lab reported. I knew almost from the start that what had happened to me would permanently change my sense of self. I'd been a surgeon who frequently did cancer surgery. Now, as I put it in the title of a book on my own experience with cancer, it was "the surgeon's turn."

Back I went to surgery, this time to have my thyroid removed completely. That experience was followed by treatment with radioactive iodine (I^{131}).

Since then, I've done O.K. Each year I visit my endocrinologist for tests (he specializes in diseases and treatment of ductless glands). Every day I give myself doses of thyroid to replace what my body can no longer manufacture. So it is that I came to take a special interest in this relatively obscure disease.

WHAT THE THYROID IS AND WHAT IT DOES

The thyroid is an endocrine (ductless) gland located in the neck below the Adam's apple. The largest of the endocrine glands, it is shaped like a butterfly, with two lateral lobes that look like wings. Each lobe is made up of many sacs or follicles lined by a single layer of cells. These cells are, if you will, the business end of the thyroid gland. They produce the thyroid hormone that is stored in the follicles. This hormone is directly involved in determining your energy level.

How much or how little of the hormone is produced is determined by another endocrine gland called the pituitary gland, located at the base of the brain. The pituitary itself gets the message to release the thyroid hormone from a feedback mechanism at the base of the brain called the hypothalamus.

The hormone itself comes from thyroglobulin, and normally is produced only by the cells in the lining of the thyroid sacs. But cancer cells can also produce thyroglobulin. That is why the recurrence of this hormone *after* the thyroid has been removed is evidence of cancer.

We said earlier that the thyroid hormone is involved in your energy level. Here is how. The thyroid gland attaches iodine in your diet to thyroglobulin. Once the conversion is complete, the new thyroid hormone works to control the rate by which your body produces protein and uses oxygen to convert food into energy. You couldn't live without it.

WHAT THYROID CANCER IS

Thyroid cancer is a disease in which the cells lining a follicle become abnormal, grow out of control, and eventually form a malignant tumor. As with any cancer, if it isn't treated early enough and effectively, it can spread locally—that is, without distant metastases—to vital structures like the trachea (windpipe), or may invade the large blood vessels of the neck and cause bleeding. The cancer can also spread by way of the bloodstream to other organs, like the lung, bones, or liver.

CAUSES OF THYROID CANCER

We know only a little about this subject. We know, for instance, that the disease is more common in whites than blacks, in women than men. But we don't know why. We also know that irradiation to the head and neck in childhood is an important risk factor. Until that fact was discovered, external beam radiation was used to treat relatively minor ailments like ringworm of the scalp, acne, and enlarged tonsils and thymus glands. People who received such treatment are at much higher risk for thyroid cancers although the cancers don't develop until many years after the treatment. If the doses were as high as 1,500 rads, the risk is thirtyfold.

Working or living near nuclear power plants may also add to

risk. So do nuclear accidents. After the Chernobyl accident cancer rates rose sharply.

Certain specific thyroid cancers appear to be genetically caused. In my own family, not only my mother but an aunt as well had tumors of the thyroid before I did.

PREVENTION

Avoiding radiation treatments in childhood is the best prevention. But these are uncommon nowadays in any case. Where cancers run in a family, genetic counseling can be of some help in that it encourages regular monitoring by means of blood tests.

Finally, we know that testing nuclear weapons releases into the atmosphere high amounts of radioactive products. Testing at the Nevada site in the 1950s exposed residents of the entire nation to I^{131}. Though individual cases of thyroid cancer cannot be traced directly to these tests, we must assume we will all be healthier without them.

DIAGNOSING THYROID CANCER

Preliminary diagnosis of thyroid cancer will be determined by palpating the neck. As in the case of breast cancer, the tumor must be at least 1 cm in size in order to be detected by the hand. This means—here again the case resembles breast cancer—there may be tumors too small to be detected by the hand.

Most small tumors in the thyroid are benign and need not be removed. Final diagnosis must be done by taking a biopsy sample and examining the tissue under a microscope. The sample is taken by needle aspiration, a nonsurgical procedure. If the tumor contains mostly benign cells, surgery isn't indicated unless the patient is suffering from discomfort because of pressure from the tumor.

If tumors are present in the sample of thyroid cells called *follic-*

ular cells, surgery is required, because in such a case only examination of the entire tumor can reveal whether cancer is present. An absolute diagnosis of follicular thyroid cancer means either that follicular cells have invaded the capsule of the tumor or that they are present in the blood vessels.

I should add that other doctors may employ additional tests to those I've described. The patient may be given a dose of low-radiation iodine (I^{131}), which, by detecting those areas of the gland that absorb the material, can distinguish between the hot and cold areas. Thyroid scans can determine whether particular areas of the thyroid are functioning or not (in our lingo, "hot" or "cold"). Cancer is more common in cold nodules.

Ultrasound tests, in which high-frequency waves are bounced off the thyroid and translated by a computer into a sonogram (picture), can distinguish between a cyst (usually benign) and a solid tumor, which may be cancerous.

Diagnosis is a process that moves from suspicion through probability to certainty. Recall that in my own case the initial diagnosis was a benign adenoma. Only after the pathologist performed a more detailed study was that diagnosis changed from benign to malignant.

Early stages of thyroid cancer produce few symptoms except the tumor or nodule itself. If the disease advances, the patient may experience a "full feeling" or tightness in the neck. Later, this will be followed by hoarseness, which means a nerve to the voice box is involved. On rare occasions, at an advanced stage, the patient may have difficulty swallowing or even breathing.

TYPES OF THYROID CANCER AND THEIR TREATMENT

Papillary Cancer
The most common of the four types of thyroid cancer is papillary, which also has the highest survival rates. Papillary thyroid cancer

involves small tumors, under 1 cm, and it is usually discovered when the thyroid is removed for some other condition. Papillary cancer is not invasive and does not involve lymph nodes. Treatment requires simple removal of the affected lobe of the thyroid. After the operation, the patient will take thyroid hormone to suppress the pituitary secretion (TSH) that may stimulate the thyroid to produce other tumors. Yearly checkups are necessary to monitor any recurrence.

The typical thyroid papillary cancer requires more extensive surgery. These cancers often will occur in several areas. In the worst cases, they may invade the trachea and esophagus, then spread to lymph nodes in the neck and eventually metastasize to the lung and other organs.

This cancer presents a special problem, in that in 7 to 18 percent of cases it recurs in the other lobe after the one lobe has been removed. Some surgeons will remove only the involved lobe and connecting isthmus and then carefully monitor the patient. Some surgeons, including myself, totally remove the thyroid gland.

This kind of case also requires removal of affected lymph nodes in the neck. These can be removed individually, in a procedure we call *cherry picking*, or by removing the fatty tissue in the neck that contains the nodes.

By removing most or all of both lobes, we have better insurance that the cancer won't recur. What thyroid tissue remains may be killed with radioactive iodine. Radioactive iodine can also control a recurrent or metastatic tumor, if all the thyroid has been removed in the original operation.

Once again, thyroid hormone will be administered as replacement therapy and to counter the TSH from the pituitary.

I have been urging radical surgery as the best approach to thyroid cancer. One additional reason I believe in it is that it allows us to use the thyroid hormone itself (thyroglobulin) as a tumor marker. If a part of the thyroid is left functioning, it will continue to secrete thyroglobulin. If all the thyroid has been removed, the presence of thyroglobulin indicates recurrent tumor. Should treatment fail at this point and the tumor comes back, it may be removed surgically.

Follicular Cancer

Follicular and papillary cancers account for 80–90 percent of all thyroid cancers. As my own case shows, follicular cancer is more difficult to diagnose than papillary cancer because the follicular cancer cells resemble those of a benign thyroid tumor, or adenoma. Positive diagnosis is possible only when the pathologist notes these cells in the covering (capsule) of the thyroid gland itself or in the blood vessels.

In many respects, my own case was typical. Because the initial pathology report pointed to a benign adenoma, the surgeon removed only a single lobe. Two days later, however, after the pathologist had time for a more thorough review, he discovered cells invading the capsule, or covering, of the tumor.

That is when the diagnosis changed to follicular carcinoma, and the surgeon had me return to surgery to remove the remainder of my thyroid gland. I was then given an iodine scan, and that revealed no metastases. This was followed by I^{131} treatment for the purpose of killing any remaining tumor, and replacement therapy to block TSH. My thyroid hormone levels were also monitored to detect any recurrence of the cancer.

Follicular cancer usually occurs in older people, and it rarely spreads to the lymph nodes. However, though papillary cancer is five times more common, more deaths result from follicular cancer. That is because, in too many cases, the diagnosis comes too late for effective treatment. The earlier follicular cancer is diagnosed, the less likely it is to have spread to distant organs such as the lungs, bones, liver, and brain. And the less the disease has spread, the better the chance of effective treatment.

Follicular cancer can also mask itself. In some cases, it forms cysts easily mistaken for anaplastic carcinoma, occurring in only 1–2 percent of thyroid cases. It can also produce excess thyroid hormones and masquerade as a hyperthyroid lesion—that is, one that produces an excess of thyroid hormone, causing a condition called *hyperthyroidism.*

A characteristic of both papillary and follicular cancer is that both can remain dormant for periods as long as fifteen to twenty years and then return. That is why some doctors advise that the thyroglobulin levels of patients who have suffered from these forms of the disease be monitored over many years, and that they also be scanned over that period. My cancer recurred seventeen years later and required removal of a lobe of the right lung.

Anaplastic Carcinoma

This third kind of thyroid cancer, *anaplastic carcinoma,* is the most malignant. Fortunately, it is rare, occurring in only 1–2 percent of all thyroid cancers, usually in patients seventy years or older. About one-third of these cases are patients who experience a recurrence of cancers that were originally papillary or follicular. We don't know why the original tumors convert to this more aggressive kind.

This tumor acts quickly and lethally. Within seven to twelve months of diagnosis, it can progressively block the trachea and erode blood vessels in the neck, with the result of massive bleeding. Symptoms include metastases to the lungs that produce fever and weakness, but patients succumb to the rapidly progressive neck problems.

The cells of this tumor are easily confused with those of lymphoma. In these cases, external radiations may be tried. But though lymphomas sometimes react favorably to radiation, it rarely is effective in the case of anaplastic carcinoma. Chemotherapy, too, may be tried, but it is rarely effective.

Medullary Carcinoma

Medullary carcinoma sometimes runs in families (20 percent of the cases, according to some researchers), sometimes not (sporadic). Medullary carcinoma produces a chemical called calcitonin, so the presence of that chemical points to the presence of the disease.

Medullary carcinoma is peculiar in that it can occur as early as two years of age or as late as eighty.

Patients with this cancer may have single or multiple tumors in the thyroid. In 15 to 20 percent of the cases, the cancer has spread to neck lymph nodes by the time it is diagnosed. Diarrhea is the most common symptom. In about 10 percent of the cases, patients have hoarseness or difficulty in swallowing. Alcohol consumption may bring on episodic flushing.

Medullary carcinoma that runs in families may be confined to the thyroid, or involve multiple endocrine glands, a syndrome called multiple endocrine neoplasia (MEN).

There are three main types of MEN: MEN 1, MEN 2A, and MEN 2B. Eash type is associated with a particular cluster of diseases. MEN 1 is associated with parathyroid tumors, pancreatic tumors, and pituitary tumors. Both MEN 2A and MEN 2B are characterized by medullary thyroid cancer and pheochromocytoma, a tumor of the adrenal gland that causes hypertension. MEN 2A is, in addition, associated with parathyroid tumors. The parathyroids are glands lying on or near the thyroid that may become overactive. If overactive, they produce high calcium levels in the bloodstream. MEN 2B is a disease cluster that includes mucosal neuromas, which may grow within the nerves of the tongue and the lips. The medullary cancer of MEN 2B is very malignant and comes at an early age. Few patients live beyond thirty or forty. Patients with MEN 2B have common characteristics: thick lips, broad noses, and, often, long, spindly arms and legs, and very flexible joints.

Families in which the MEN syndrome is inherited often have common features. Technically, we define that type as having an *autosomal dominant feature*. (If one parent has an abnormal gene and the other parent a normal gene, there is a 50 percent chance each child will inherit the abnormal gene, and therefore the dominant trait.) Because 50 percent of the children of these families will develop the tumor, genetic counseling for them is important. The counselor would make clear the risk and would discuss such options as testing the fetus, abortion, testing children, and so on.

High calcitonin levels in these cases must be taken as evidence of medullary thyroid cancer, whether or not the examining physician can feel tumors. In such cases, the thyroid should be removed entirely (*thyroidectomy*). The pathologist will likely find small, multiple tumors in the thyroid tissues. This surgery should be done even on children if the calcitonin is elevated.

Further, such genetically targeted patients should be checked for hypertension and the adrenal tumor (*pheochromocytoma*). If such a tumor is present, it must be taken care of first, lest these patients suffer a hypertension crisis under anesthesia.

Initial treatment for medullary cancer is surgical removal of the thyroid gland, as well as surrounding lymph nodes. Chemotherapy and radiation are not very effective. Seventy to 80 percent of people who have had successful surgery (that is, with all malignant cells removed) live at least ten years after diagnosis.

Medullary cancer does not respond to radioactive iodine and is relatively insensitive to external x-ray therapy. Surgery offers the only chance for cure. If metastasis occurs after surgery, removal of the tumor may help decrease the symptoms of diarrhea and flushing. Chemotherapy with doxorubicin and other agents may provide remission.

THE COMPLICATIONS OF THYROID SURGERY

As in all surgery, complications can include:

- Bleeding
- Infection
- Heart problems, and more.

But there are two major complications of thyroid surgery the surgeon must especially be on guard against. The first is injury to the nerves that control the muscles of the voice box. If these are injured, chronic hoarseness and difficulty in breathing occurs. Second, removal of, or damage to, the parathyroid glands will cause a decrease in calcium, which results in muscle spasms.

In summary, cancer of the thyroid gland is the most common cancer of the *endocrine glands* (glands that produce hormones). It usually presents as a palpable tumor in the neck. Patients often discover such tumors as I did, while shaving, and while applying makeup. Such a tumor needs immediate attention. If you find one, see your doctor at once.

Remember, during the period from 1995 to 1999, African-American women died at nearly twice the rate of whites.

IN A NUTSHELL

Incidence:
In the United States in 2006, estimates show thyroid cancer diagnosed in over 30,000 men and women.

Cause:
- X-ray treatment to neck in children for benign conditions (thymus, acne, and so on)
- Genetic (familial).

Prevention:
Avoid x-ray treatment for benign conditions.

Diagnosis:
- Be alert to a lump in your neck.
- Your doctor will do a biopsy, check for "cold" nodules on scan, and check for elevated calcitonin levels (which can indicate medullary cancer).

Treatment:
Thyroidectomy (total or partial removal of thyroid).

Prognosis:
- Papillary: good to excellent with early treatment
- Follicular: good if treated early with careful follow-up
- Medullary: fair to good with early treatment
- Undifferentiated: very poor.

TEN

Uterine Endometrial Cancer

WHEN MARIE ALLEN first began experiencing abnormal, excessive, vaginal bleeding at the age of thirty-eight, during her menstruation periods, she thought she could explain her condition away. One friend of hers had experienced such bleeding, only to learn that she was having a miscarriage. Another friend learned that her bleeding was caused by *fibroids* (tumors in the wall of the uterus or womb), and her symptoms vanished as menopause approached. So Marie waited for her bleeding to vanish.

Instead, it continued. She grew weaker and more pale, until she knew she could delay no longer. Her family physician found her to be anemic. "There are a thousand possible causes for anemia," he told her, "but since you are bleeding, I think it's best that you see a gynecologist."

A gynecologist is a doctor who specializes in the pelvic diseases of women, and Marie visited the one her family doctor recommended. The test was simple enough: the gynecologist inserted a tube into her vagina and took a sample. A week later, Marie got a call from the doctor. She had cancer of the uterus, and she needed immediate transfusion. "After that," the doctor told her, "we can start treating you."

Marie's condition was complicated by the fact that she had diabetes and hypertension and she was obese. Since each of those conditions is a risk factor, hers didn't promise to be a simple case.

ENDOMETRIAL CANCER IN BLACK WOMEN

Black women are less likely to get endometrial cancer than white women, but are more likely to die of it (see Figure 12 page 138). One reason for this discrepancy may be that black women are less likely to be diagnosed and treated early. Another is that, when treated, too often they receive different, and often less effective, types of treatment than white women because:

- Poverty can make access to health facilities difficult.
- Lack of insurance—obviously related to poverty—can deny access.
- Racial discrimination, pure and simple, can deny our women appropriate medical treatment.

While we don't know the cause of endometrial cancer, we do know some of the risk factors. Keep in mind that you can have these risk factors without having cancer.

The National Cancer Institute lists these risk factors for endometrial cancer:

- Age. Cancer of the uterus occurs mostly in women over age fifty.
- Endometrial hyperplasia. The risk of uterine cancer is higher if a woman has endometrial hyperplasia.
- Hormone replacement therapy (HRT). HRT is used to control the symptoms of menopause, to prevent osteoporosis (thinning of the bones), and to reduce the risk of heart disease or stroke.

- Women who use estrogen without progesterone have an increased risk of uterine cancer. Long-term use and large doses of estrogen seem to increase this risk. Women who use a combination of estrogen and progesterone have a lower risk of uterine cancer than women who use estrogen alone. The progesterone protects the uterus.
- Women should discuss the benefits and risks of HRT with their doctor. Also, having regular checkups while taking HRT may improve the chance that the doctor will find uterine cancer at an early stage, if it does develop.

- Obesity and related conditions. The body makes some of its estrogen in fatty tissue. That's why obese women are more likely than thin women to have higher levels of estrogen in their bodies. High levels of estrogen may be the reason that obese women have an increased risk of developing uterine cancer. The risk of this disease is also higher in women with diabetes or high blood pressure (conditions that occur in many obese women).
- Tamoxifen. Women taking the drug tamoxifen to prevent or treat breast cancer have an increased risk of uterine cancer. This risk appears to be related to the estrogenlike effect of this drug on the uterus. Doctors monitor women taking tamoxifen for possible signs or symptoms of uterine cancer. The benefits of tamoxifen in the treatment of breast cancer outweighs the risk of developing other cancers. Still, each woman is different. Any woman considering taking tamoxifen should discuss with the doctor her personal and family medical history and her concerns.
- White women are more likely than African-American women to get uterine cancer.
- Colorectal cancer. Women who have had an inherited form of colorectal cancer have a higher risk of developing uterine cancer than other women.

Other risk factors are related to how long a woman's body is exposed to estrogen. Women who have no children, begin menstru-

FIGURE 12

SEER INCIDENCE AND U.S. DEATH RATES,[†] 1975–2002

Corpus and Uterus, NOS Cancer, by Age and Race

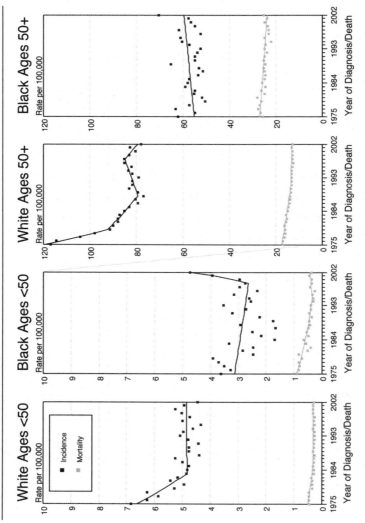

+ Source: SEER 9 areas and NCHS public use data file for the total US. Rates are age-adjusted to the 2000 US Std Population (19 age groups - Census P25-1103). Regression lines are calculated using the Joinpoint Regression Program Version 3.0, April 2005, National Cancer Institute.

Surveillance, Epidemiology, and End Results (SEER) Program (www.seer.cancer.gov) SEER*Stat Database: Incidence - SEER 9 Regs Public-Use, Nov 2004 Sub (1973-2002), National Cancer Institute, DCCPS, Surveillance Research Program, Cancer Statistics Branch, released April 2005, based on the November 2004 submission.

FIGURE 13

SEER INCIDENCE AND U.S. DEATH RATES,[†] 1975–2002

Corpus and Uterus, NOS Cancer, by Age and Race

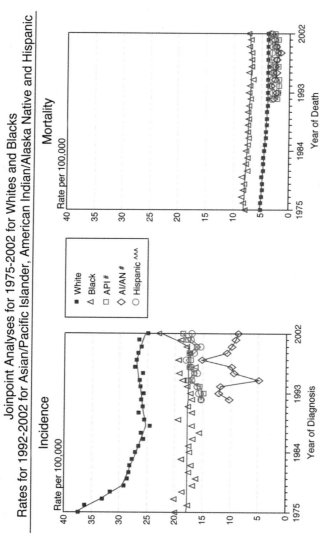

Joinpoint Analyses for 1975–2002 for Whites and Blacks
Rates for 1992–2002 for Asian/Pacific Islander, American Indian/Alaska Native and Hispanic

+ Source: Incidence data for whites and blacks is from the SEER 9 areas (San Francisco, Connecticut, Detroit, Hawaii, Iowa, New Mexico, Seattle, Utah, Atlanta). Incidence data for Asian/Pacific Islanders, American Indian/Alaska Natives and Hispanics is from the SEER 13 Areas (SEER 9 Areas, San Jose-Monterey, Los Angeles, Alaska Native Registry and Rural Georgia). Mortality data is from NCHS public use data file for the total US.
Rates are age-adjusted to the 2000 US Std Population (19 age groups - Census P25-1103).
Regression lines for whites and blacks are calculated using the Joinpoint Regression Program Version 3.0, April 2005, National Cancer Institute.
API = Asian/Pacific Islander. AI/AN = American Indian/Alaska Native.
^^ Hispanic is not mutually exclusive from Whites, Blacks, Asian/Pacific Islanders, and American Indians/Alaska Natives. Incidence data for Hispanics excludes cases from Detroit, Hawaii, Alaska Native Registry and Rural Georgia. Mortality data for Hispanics excludes cases from Connecticut, Maine, Maryland, Minnesota, Oklahoma, New Hampshire, New York, North Dakota, and Vermont.

Surveillance, Epidemiology, and End Results (SEER) Program (www.seer.cancer.gov) SEER*Stat Database: Incidence - SEER 9 Regs Public-Use, Nov 2004 Sub (1973–2002), National Cancer Institute, DCCPS, Surveillance Research Program, Cancer Statistics Branch, released April 2005, based on the November 2004 submission.

ation at a very young age, or enter menopause late in life are exposed to estrogen longer and have a higher risk.

Women with known risk factors and those who are concerned about uterine cancer should ask their doctor about the symptoms to watch for and how often to have checkups. The doctor's advice will be based on the woman's age, medical history, and other factors.

ANATOMY AND FUNCTION OF THE UTERUS

The uterus, or womb, is a pear-shaped organ located in the pelvis (lower abdomen). More specifically, it is located between the bladder in front and the rectum behind. The larger, upper part of the uterus is called the body, the lower part, or neck and outlet, is called the cervix. The body has an inner lining called the *endometrium*. It is from this lining that cancer of the uterus arises. (Cancer of the cervix will be discussed in the next chapter.)

The function of the uterus is to house the fetus during its development. The cervix provides an exit for the fetus during its delivery.

CAUSES OF ENDOMETRIAL CANCER

As is often the case with cancer, though we can't identify specific causes, we *can* identify risk factors:

- Prolonged exposure to estrogens may be the key. Women who begin menstruating at an early age, or who have a late menopause, or who have few or no children, are more likely than other groups to develop endometrial cancer. So are obese women, especially if they are also diabetics. Insulin works like estrogen as a growth stimulant for cancer cells.
- Genetic factors may also play a role.
- Endometrial cancer also occurs in families with a strong history of colon cancer. This syndrome is called hereditary non-

polyposis colorectal caner (HNPCC). It results from mutations in genes that are responsible for repairing damaged DNA. Once these repair genes are themselves damaged, cancers develop.

PREVENTION OF ENDOMETRIAL CANCER

Obviously, no woman can manipulate her genes to enhance P53 activity, although the day may come when medical science can do that for her. Until that day, however, black women do have some control over their destiny. What is required is very simple:

- Avoid obesity and increase fiber intake. Those two steps will reduce the reabsorption of estrogens and reduce your likelihood of developing endometrial cancer (as well as breast cancer).
- Eat lots of fresh fruit and vegetables and, as often as you can, substitute fish, with its healing oils, for meat, with its dangerous fat.

Be aware also that the use of estrogen replacement therapy during menopause can cause a tenfold increase in uterine cancer and seems to increase the risk of breast cancer. According to a study published in the *New England Journal of Medicine* (1995), the combination of progestin with estrogen protects against uterine cancer but seems to increase the risk of breast cancer.

DIAGNOSIS

A history of abnormal uterine bleeding is usually the initial complaint. But there are other more common and less dangerous causes of vaginal bleeding. In black women, fibroids (a benign, muscular tumor of the uterus) are especially common.

Another cause of such bleeding is a precancerous lesion caused by a condition called *hyperplasia*—a benign overproduction of cells. This condition tends to occur at an early age. It can be controlled by medication or, in extreme cases, hysterectomy.

In most cases, your doctor will perform:

- A pelvic exam
- A Pap test
- A biopsy procedure.

Final diagnosis of endometrial cancer requires biopsy by suction or *curetting* (scraping the inside of the uterus with a metal loop called a *curette*), a simple procedure.

TREATMENT

Treatment of endometrial uterine cancer depends on the stage. As always, staging of endometrial cancer in strict medical terms can be complicated. The simpler system recommended for patients is the FIGO system, with modifications:

- Stage I: Confined to uterine lining and half of muscular wall.
- Stage II: Extension of tumor to lining of cervix.
- Stage III: Tumor invades outer layer of uterus or tubes and ovary or vagina or lymph nodes.
- Stage IV: Tumor invades bladder or intestines or distal spread.

The treatment of a stage I lesion is usually total removal of the uterus, tubes and ovaries. To assure that the cancer has not spread to other organs, including lymph nodes, careful examination of the internal organs is done at the time of surgery. Gynecologists trained in cancer management, known as *gyn-oncologists,* are the experts in this area and should be consulted before starting on a treatment course.

Well-trained ob-gyn physicians frequently do hysterectomies for nonmalignant conditions. A diagnosis of cancer requires a different approach, with added expertise. I would recommend consulting such a specialist before treatment.

Surgical treatment involves removing the uterus, tubes and ovaries through the abdomen. A major decision made by the surgeon is whether to remove the pelvic lymph nodes. This entails increased surgical risks and should be done only in situations in which the lymph nodes are thought to be positive for the cancer.

About 9 percent of patients with early-stage endometrial cancer will be found to have lymph node metastasis. Many of these patients can be successfully treated with radiation; therefore they do not need to undergo the complicated risky procedure of removing the pelvic lymph nodes.

Radiation therapy is critical to treatment in those patients with advanced stage I, or greater, disease. This treatment helps to destroy any hidden metastases to the lymph nodes or the vagina.

Radical removal of *all* pelvic organs, including uterus, bladder, and rectum, is seldom justified. It rarely improves prognosis.

If peritoneal washings (washings of the membrane lining of the abdominal cavity) reveal malignant cells, external radiation or chemotherapy is the appropriate treatment.

Beyond stage II, the patient's outlook is not good. In such patients, x-ray treatment is better than no treatment. But removal of the uterus, fallopian tubes, and ovaries is the best course.

Stage II and stage III patients should have preoperative x-ray therapy followed by radical hysterectomy, including tubes and ovaries. If the patient is a poor surgical risk, primary x-ray may be given although the results are not as good as when surgery is done.

Recurrent or far-advanced tumors will also respond to tamoxifen, raloxifene, or progestin therapy in 30 percent of cases. Drugs like doxorubicin and platinum may also be of value.

Tumors with less malignant cells contain cells with progesterone receptors and respond best to antiestrogen drugs like raloxifene.

PROGNOSIS

Prognosis is excellent at the early stage. The fact that heavy uterine bleeding is an early symptom is an advantage. This is not a cancer that conceals its symptoms until it is too late to treat effectively.

This means that, upon any sign of such abnormal bleeding, you need to see your doctor. Insist on a pelvic exam, Pap smear, and a clear diagnosis. If you are not satisfied, seek a second opinion, or even a third. Don't rely on the opinions of friends and relatives, and don't rest until your doctor gives you a clear opinion of your condition.

Endometrial cancer is a highly treatable disease as long as the patient is diagnosed in time and is given prompt treatment.

As we said earlier, black women are more likely than white women to die of endometrial cancer. The National Cancer Data Base (NCDB) reports that the kinds of tumors found in black women are less likely to be glandular tumors—called *adenocarcinoma,* which have a more favorable prognosis.

Endometrial cancer is a curable disease as long as the patient is diagnosed in time and is given prompt treatment.

But there is another kind of difference still more worrisome. The NCDB also reports that "nine percent of the African American patients did not receive any cancer-directed treatment compared with four percent of the White patients, and they were treated less often at every stage of diagnosis." If this were simply a symptom of economic discrimination, it would be bad enough. But the report goes on to say that "income generally had no effect on whether treatment was provided."

I will speak further, in Chapter 21, on the need for equality in health care, about the kind of persistent problem this report indisputably identifies. Obviously, in matters of health, as in too many others, not all women appear, in the minds of their doctors, to be created equal.

For the black woman there's a lesson to be drawn from this. If you walk into your doctor's office with knowledge about your condition and about the treatments appropriate to it, you are far more likely to get the careful diagnosis and, if needed, the treatment that you need. On the basis of such information as we provide here, prepare a list of questions before you visit your doctor. If he or she is unwilling to answer them, find another doctor. It's as simple as that.

If your doctor is unwilling to answer your questions, find another doctor.

It's important that you ask your questions clearly and politely. Doctors are human, all too human, and if you come on harshly, they will probably react in kind. But get your questions asked and get them answered.

Here are a few examples:

Ask your questions clearly and politely.

- What tests will I need in order to find out if this excessive bleeding I've been having is caused by endometrial cancer or by something less serious?
- (After the diagnosis) Please tell me something about the treatment you propose for my stage I (or II, III, or IV) endometrial cancer.
- (If treatment involves total removal of the uterus and ovaries) What will be the long-range implications of this loss? And please tell me why, since this loss is considerable, that it's the wise choice for me.
- Do you recommend radiation therapy after the operation?
- Are there other postoperative therapies that I'll need?
- What possible complication can result from surgery and x-ray treatment?
- How long before I can return to work, and to my normal life?

MARIE ALLEN'S CASE: THE AFTERMATH

Marie Allen proved to be an excellent patient. With her active coop-eration, we got her diabetes and hypertension treated and con-trolled. After being given 3 pints of blood, she had her uterus, tubes, and ovaries removed. The operation confirmed what the diagnosis pointed to: she had a stage II lesion.

Marie is doing very well two years after the operation. She con-tinues on her weight-reduction diet and raloxifene.

AN URGENT WORD OF ADVICE

One of the most important things I have to say to you on the sub-ject of endometrial cancer is that black women must learn to accept the necessity of having their uterus and ovaries removed when the diagnosis requires. Yes, a woman loses her ability to menstruate, and therefore her ability to bear children after such an operation. But she does *not* lose sexual desire, performance, or sexuality in any respect except that of childbearing.

I write as a man, with the knowledge that no man can under-stand fully the fear and avoidance a woman will feel if she's told that she needs such an operation, nor the psychological impact such treatment may have. But I've known too many women who, when they began to experience excessive bleeding, went into all the acro-batics of denial. In some cases, the result was that when they were finally diagnosed, it was too late to save them.

That's why I'll repeat the central lesson of this chapter: *if you suf-fer abnormal vaginal bleeding, see your physician at once. Only a doc-tor can determine whether or not the cause of the bleeding is cancer.*

IN A NUTSHELL

Incidence:

Endometrial cancer, with some 40,000 new cases each year, is the most common cancer of the female genital organs. Although black women are 3.3 percent less likely to contract endometrial cancer than white women, they are nearly two times more likely to die of it.

Cause:
- Excessive exposure to estrogens
- Risk factors include obesity, diabetes, hypertension.

Prevention:
- Reduce exposure to estrogens.
- Correct risk factors.
- Go on a high-fiber, low-fat diet to counteract estrogen absorption in intestines.
- Get hysterectomy if you are diagnosed with extensive hyperplasia.

Diagnosis:
- Be alert to abnormal vaginal bleeding (excessive menstrual bleeding or bleeding between periods).
- Endometrial biopsy.

Treatment:
- Hysterectomy if stage I
- Hysterectomy and removal of both tubes and ovaries with or without x-ray therapy and chemotherapy if cancer is in stages II through IV
- Pre- or postoperative radiation is usually given to treat known or unknown lymph node involvement of metastasis to the vagina.

Prognosis:
- Good for stages I and II
- Progressively poorer in stages III and IV.

ELEVEN

Uterine Cervical Cancer

LOLA'S CASE

IN THE BATHROOM ONE NIGHT after intense lovemaking, Lola Austin noticed vaginal spotting, but she thought nothing about it. She'd had a Pap smear after all, and it was normal. So Lola pretended to herself that nothing was going on. It was only when her lover, Malcolm, noticed that the spotting had gone on for several months that he could persuade her to see a doctor. "Sure, it's probably nothing, Lola," he said. "But that Pap smear you took—that was five years ago. You need another one now, and while you're at it, get a good examination."

Malcolm had to prod her once or twice more before she finally made an appointment and got her exam. When Dr. Arnold called her to come in for a report on the Pap smear, she was uneasy. With good reason, it turned out. "I'm sorry to tell you this, Lola," he said in his office, "but the Pap smear came back positive. We'll need to biopsy your cervix."

Lola was uneasy about the doctor's recommendation, so she asked some questions.

"Since you already have the results of the Pap smear, why do you need to do this?"

Dr. Arnold explained: "The Pap smear gives us only a few cells to examine. It's accurate, as far as it goes, but it's a little like looking at a few scattered pieces of a jigsaw puzzle and trying to guess the whole picture. The biopsy brings us closer to the whole picture: it shows us how the cells are connected to each other. It also shows how they are attached to a membrane—if they are attached. So we come away with a much fuller picture of the situation."

"O.K.," Lola, said. "But I have another question. I'm afraid of pain. How bad will this hurt?"

"That's a good question, Lola. Some patients are embarrassed to ask it. The fact is that the cervix isn't very sensitive, so there's very little pain, and the procedure takes only a few minutes. There may be a little discomfort, and it may feel a little undignified—but, as I say, the whole thing is over in a few minutes."

"O.K.," said Lola, "let's do it."

Unfortunately, the biopsy confirmed the Pap smear finding. Lola had cervical cancer, a malignancy that occurs at the lower outlet of the uterus.

Lola was one of an estimated 10,370 women each year who are diagnosed with this disease. About 3,710 of them will die of it. Though cervical cancer ranks third among cancers of the female genital system, after endometrial and ovarian cancer, it's a cancer that hits black women hard. *Nearly 25 percent more black women than white women are likely to be diagnosed with the disease, and of those who are diagnosed, black women are two to three times more likely to die of it.*

Cervical cancer hits black women hard.

THE IMPORTANCE OF PAP TESTS

We've said this before but must say it again—and again: not all cancer can be prevented, but short of not getting cancer at all, the best option is to get it detected as early as possible. In the case of cervical cancer, prevention means getting an annual Pap smear. Had Lola known this, and done it, her problem would have been caught earlier, and the likelihood of successful treatment and cure would have been much better.

Pap smears dramatically reduce mortality rates from cervical cancer.

Indeed, regular Pap smears, more than any other cancer screening, have dramatically reduced mortality rates from cervical cancer. Before this test came into wide use (in 1943), women with cervical cancer did not see a doctor until the cancer was obvious—and obvious often meant it was untreatable. Regular Pap smears can detect such early warning signs as:

- Lesions of the cervix, which, though not malignant, can lead to malignancy
- Dysplasia, or cell changes that, though not in themselves cancerous, may point to cancer
- Carcinoma in-situ, which is to say, a cancer that has not yet begun to spread.

Conditions like these, caught early, can be treated by laser or cone removal. Cone removal, usually done under anesthesia, involves the removal with a knife of a small cone of tissue.

CAUSES AND PREVENTION

Strictly speaking, it's rarely possible to connect a specific cancer with a specific cause. Instead, we speak of risk factors such as being in generally poor health conditions, living a risky lifestyle, or having been exposed to toxins, which can make an individual vulnerable to a particular disease. In the case of cervical cancer, the risk factors are these:

FIGURE 14

SEER INCIDENCE AND U.S. DEATH RATES, [†] 1975–2005

Cervix Uteri Cancer, by Age and Race

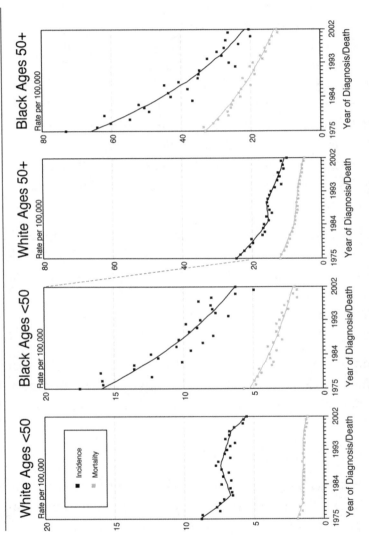

+ Source: SEER 9 areas and NCHS public use data file for the total US. Rates are age-adjusted to the 2000 US Std Population (19 age groups - Census P25-1103). Regression lines are calculated using the Joinpoint Regression Program Version 3.0, April 2005, National Cancer Institute.

Surveillance, Epidemiology, and End Results (SEER) Program (www.seer.cancer.gov) SEER*Stat Database: Incidence - SEER 9 Regs Public-Use, Nov 2004 Sub (1973-2002), National Cancer Institute, DCCPS, Surveillance Research Program, Cancer Statistics Branch, released April 2005, based on the November 2004 submission.

SEER INCIDENCE AND US DEATH RATES,[†] 1975–2005

Cervix Uteri Cancer

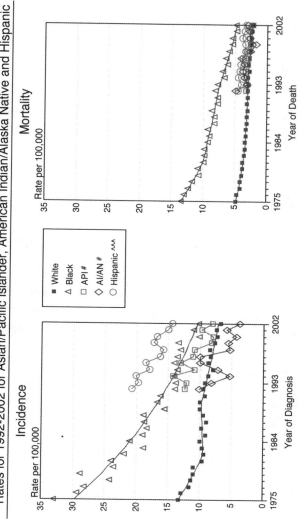
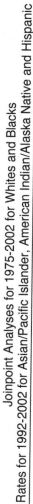

Joinpoint Analyses for 1975-2002 for Whites and Blacks
Rates for 1992-2002 for Asian/Pacific Islander, American Indian/Alaska Native and Hispanic

† Source: Incidence data for whites and blacks is from the SEER 9 areas (San Francisco, Connecticut, Detroit, Hawaii, Iowa, New Mexico, Seattle, Utah, Atlanta). Incidence data for Asian/Pacific Islanders, American Indian/Alaska Natives and Hispanics is from the SEER 13 Areas (SEER 9 Areas, San Jose-Monterey, Los Angeles, Alaska Native Registry and Rural Georgia). Mortality data is from NCHS public use data file for the total US.
Rates are age-adjusted to the 2000 US Std Population (19 age groups - Census P25-1103).
Regression lines for whites and blacks are calculated using the Joinpoint Regression Program Version 3.0, April 2005, National Cancer Institute.
API = Asian/Pacific Islander. AI/AN = American Indian/Alaska Native.
^^^ Hispanic is not mutually exclusive from Whites, Blacks, Asian/Pacific Islanders, and American Indians/Alaska Natives. Incidence data for Hispanics excludes cases from Detroit, Hawaii, Alaska Native Registry and Rural Georgia. Mortality data for Hispanics excludes cases from Connecticut, Maine, Maryland, Minnesota, Oklahoma, New Hampshire, New York, North Dakota, and Vermont.

Surveillance, Epidemiology, and End Results (SEER) Program (www.seer.cancer.gov) SEER*Stat Database: Incidence - SEER 9 Regs Public-Use, Nov 2004 Sub (1973-2002), National Cancer Institute, DCCPS, Surveillance Research Program, Cancer Statistics Branch, released April 2005, based on the November 2004 submission.

- Sexual activity in early adolescence, early pregnancy, multiple sexual partners—all these possibly related to trauma to the cervix
- Human papilloma virus, which is found in precancerous lesions, and which is more common in blacks
- HIV virus
- Herpes simplex virus
- Tobacco use.

These risk factors themselves suggest the best means of prevention:

- Don't have multiple sex partners.
- Don't have intercourse during adolescence.
- Don't have intercourse without a condom.
- Don't get pregnant during adolescence.
- Don't use tobacco or be exposed to other people's tobacco smoke.

Finally, avoid Lola's error. She believed, mistakenly, that one normal Pap smear five years ago guaranteed her freedom from developing cervical cancer. It didn't. The test should be done each year, in connection with a pelvic examination.

It's simply a question of caring enough about yourself:

- Take charge of your own sexuality by being careful of whom you sleep with.
- Get a pap smear.
- Get treatment if needed.

DIAGNOSIS

Early detection means better likelihood of effective treatment and cure. Where, as in Lola's case, the patient herself discovers symptoms, these will usually be vaginal spotting, particularly after intercourse or douching. If this occurs, see your doctor immediately.

Besides taking a Pap smear, the physician will apply an acid solution to the cervix. When the acid solution dries up, abnormal areas of the cervix will be seen.

TREATMENT

If the doctor finds that the area under examination *isn't* cancerous, but precancerous, the area can be treated by loop excision (the loop is a wire cutting device) or laser.

If the disease proves to be widespread and "of a high grade" (that is, very malignant), your doctor may recommend a hysterectomy. Hysterectomy may provide a complete cure.

Obviously, hysterectomy is a radical treatment. Some women, especially if they are older, may take this in stride. For others, it may seem an assault on their femininity. To undergo a hysterectomy can be an agonizing choice. But sometimes, when it's a question of life or death, we may find acceptable an option that earlier seemed unthinkable. The essential thing is that this operation can allow the woman to get on with her life instead of being stopped in her tracks by disease.

We have staked out two extremes: (1) conventional medical treatment in cases where there's no evidence of cancer but where there are precancerous areas, and (2) treatment of cases where the cancer is extensive and aggressive. Let us say a few words more about conventional treatment. Then we can consider other ways of thinking about cervical cancer.

As in all kinds of cancer, treatment of cervical cancer depends on the stage of the disease. The staging system for cervical cancer, called FIGO, looks like this in simplified form:

- Stage 0: Carcinoma in-situ (that is, precancerous cells rather than frank or invasive cancer).
- Stage 1: Tumor is confined to cervix.
- Stage II: Tumor has spread to upper two-thirds of the vagina with or without a lateral spread part way to the pelvic wall.

- Stage III: Tumor has spread to lower one-third of vagina or spread laterally to pelvic wall or ureters are (tubes from kidney to bladder) blocked.
- Stage IV: Tumor has spread outside reproductive tract, whether to bladder or rectum or more distant organs.

Stage 0 is a precancerous stage. From our viewpoint, it is also the critical stage. It is here that a precancerous condition can be detected and treated. Indeed, it is our belief that, through annual Pap smears and early treatment, where necessary, cervical cancer may be virtually eliminated.

When actual cancer—doctors call it *frank* or *invasive* cancer—develops, as you know, the first sign is, in most cases, spotting or bleeding. Effective treatment is still possible at this stage, but it's essential that the patient immediately come in for a checkup. By delaying that checkup by several months, Lola allowed the cancer to spread, and hurt her chances for full recovery.

When her biopsy report came in, she learned that her cancer was stage I and treatable. (These 10 to 15 percent are cases classified as stage I *before* surgery that, after surgery, turn out to have invaded the lymph nodes.) Although Lola's disease was still at an early stage, the aggressive nature of cervical cancer required that she get decisive treatment. Her lesion—that is, cancer—confined to her cervix, could be treated with radiation.

More effective treatments are hysterectomy or radical hysterectomy. (Radical hysterectomy includes the removal of nearby lymph nodes.) The effectiveness of such treatment depends on the stage of the cancer. In some cases, radiation treatment, in the form of cesium implant, precedes surgery.

Early in stage II, lesions in the cervix can be treated by x-ray or by cesium implants, which are removed after a few days. But such treatment destroys the activity of the ovaries. For that reason, women who still want to bear children may wish to avoid it. An argument for surgical treatment is that, except in the case of radical hysterectomy, it leaves the ovaries unaffected.

For stage III and stage IV cervical cancers, surgery is ruled out. The cancer has spread to the pelvic wall and not all of it can be removed by surgery. X-ray treatment is the strongest alternative. While the survival rate for stage I cancers is 80%–85%, for stage II it is 60%–80% when the upper part of the vagina is involved, and for stage III 30%–50%. In stage IV, when the cancer has invaded the bladder or rectum and has spread beyond the pelvis, the survival rate is only 14%. Five-year survival rate falls to 20%–25%. *African-American women are almost two-and-a-half times more likely than white women to die of cervical cancer.*

In extreme cases, the tumor spreads along the aorta (the large blood vessel in the abdomen that carries blood to the intestines and legs). When that happens, chances are that the cancer has spread widely and is probably incurable.

Because such cancers can recur even after surgery, x-ray is a desirable follow-up treatment. It's also more or less the only treatment available if the cancer comes back after surgery has been performed. Sometimes, a small spot of cancer *can* be removed by surgery at this stage. But generally, one must put one's faith in x-ray.

In certain cases, surgery more radical than hysterectomy can be helpful. Such surgery is called *pelvic exenteration,* and it involves the removal of all the major organs in the pelvis, including the rectum and bladder. Sometimes such operations are moderated, and leave the rectum in place. In such cases, a substitute bladder is created out of the colon. Such operations are among the most difficult that a surgeon performs.

Through Pap smears and early treatment, cervical cancer may be virtually eliminated.

We don't pretend that it's easy to throw a rosy light over any of this. That's why it's so important that you do what you can to prevent yourself from getting this cancer, or any other. We're happy to say that African-American women have become more aware of the threat posed by cervical cancer. The number of African-American women who have a Pap test has improved to 84.1 percent.

Remember, if cervical cancer is detected in stage I or early in stage II, prognosis is quite good. In stages III and IV, prognosis becomes very bad. Regular annual Pap smears and careful follow-up can ensure that you will not be the victim of a stage III or stage IV cervical cancer.

There's also a new test that holds much promise. The human papilloma virus (HPV), as we said earlier, is found in conjunction with many cases of cervical cancer, and can be considered a cause of it. (This is a good reason for having sex with only one person or for using a condom.) Because HPV can be detected by testing for its DNA, an HPV test is now possible. It's simple enough: the doctor or nurse or even the patient herself simply uses a swab to obtain material from the cervix. Care must be taken to ensure that the swab does not miss the targeted area.

Dr. Thomas Wright of Columbia University Medical Center has done pioneer studies on the HPV virus and cervical cancer and believes that it is a good screening test. If the test comes back positive, a biopsy of the cervix is needed. But because this test *can* miss its target, we believe that it should be used along with a Pap smear. Continue to see your doctor for an annual pelvic exam and Pap test, and ask him or her if you should also get the HPV test.

Although early detection is essential, prevention should also be an essential part of your protection plan. Of all the risk factors for cancer, smoking is the most preventable. The National Cancer Institute reports that smoking causes 87 percent of lung cancer death, and for 30 percent of all cancer deaths in the United States. "Tobacco is the most preventable cause of premature death in the United States and is responsible for about 30 percent of all cancer deaths"—including cervical cancer. African Americans are smoking less than they used to, but they still smoke too much—more than white and other ethnic populations. They also have a high incidence of smoking-related illnesses.

Diets high in fruits and vegetables, most researchers agree, help fend off a variety of cancers. Dieticians urge at least five servings a day of fruits and vegetables. That's a lot, to be sure, but it's just a matter of changing habits and learning to reach for a piece of fruit or a handful of raisins or a celery stalk when your first impulse is to reach for a Big Mac or pork skins.

Finally, we know that exercise helps prevent colon cancer and breast cancer. Though we can't say with confidence that it also helps prevent cervical cancer, there's a commonsense element here we can all understand. People who take care of themselves, give some proper regard to their bodies, are at least a little careful about what they eat and drink, and are willing to stretch their limbs and get their heart pumping daily are likely to be strong and vital people. And strong and vital people are less likely to get sick than flabby, wheezing ones. We think it's as simple as that.

LOLA TODAY

Lola was in to see us just a month ago for her follow-up exam. Hysterectomy and follow-up x-rays seem to have done the trick.

"I'll tell you, doctor," Lola said, "I *know* that I'm a lucky woman. I just wasn't taking care of my body the way it deserves. Now I tell my friends, so often they're tired of listening, 'Get your annual Pap smears. No excuse not to.' They're tired of listening, but they hear me. Lucky as I am, both my friends and I know that I'd have been luckier still if I'd got my own annual Pap smears before the cancer really got going."

IN A NUTSHELL

Incidence:
Each year 10,370 women are diagnosed with this disease. Some 3,710 of them will die of it.

Cause:
Multiple sex partners, early sexual activity, early pregnancy, HIV, human papilloma virus.

Prevention:
Get annual Pap smears; avoid multiple sex partners; use condoms; have precancerous lesions removed; and keep yourself healthy by not smoking, eating right, and exercising regularly.

Diagnosis:
Pap smears and biopsy; HPV test; or, if the condition goes on too long, vaginal bleeding or spotting.

Treatment:
Early cervical cancer will require x-ray therapy or hysterectomy. In the late stages, x-ray therapy is the treatment. If the cancer recurs, either x-ray treatment or exenteration (which, you recall, involves the removal of major organs in the pelvis) will be needed.

Prognosis:
- Good for stages I and II
- Progressively worse for states II and IV.

TWELVE

Ovarian Cancer

I KNOW MORE ABOUT ovarian cancer than I would like to. Some years ago, at the end of a wonderful vacation I'd spent with my mother in Florida, she asked me to examine a hard small knot in her navel. The moment I saw it I knew what it was: such knots are the most apparent symptoms of metastatic cancer in women.

I brought my mother back to Indianapolis so she could be treated at my hospital. The biopsy performed there pointed to cancer of the ovary. Back then, no very effective therapy was available for an ovarian cancer as advanced as hers. We tried chemotherapy, but it did little good. My mother survived for six months, depressed and ill from the disease and the treatment. Nothing is harder for a doctor than to see a patient slip away while he is powerless to change the grim course of a disease. I hardly have to say how hard it was for me that in this case my patient was my mother.

ANATOMY AND PHYSIOLOGY OF THE OVARY

The ovaries are two small, white organs in the pelvis attached to the uterus by two ducts that carry the eggs, or *ova*, produced by the ovary, to the uterus (womb) to be fertilized if a sperm is present in the cavity of the uterus.

Ovaries produce the female hormones estrogen and progesterone.

As small as they are, the ovaries do much to make the person. They produce the female hormones estrogen and progesterone. These hormones, in turn, are responsible for a woman's secondary sexual features: enlarged breasts, wide hips, and appropriately placed deposits of subcutaneous fats.

WHY OVARIAN CANCER IS HARD TO TREAT

Ovarian cancer is the fifth most common cause of cancer deaths in women, ranking behind lung, breast, colon and pancreatic cancer, in that order. Even among cancers that attack the womb, ovarian cancer is not the most typical. Cancer of the cervix (mouth of the womb) and cancer of the lining of the uterus or endometrium are far more common, but they cause far fewer deaths.

Ovarian cancer presents one central problem. Unlike the other cancers I've spoken of, ovarian cancer pro-

Ovarian cancer produces few early symptoms.

duces few early symptoms. All too often, as in my mother's case, by the time the patient notices anything wrong, the cancer has already begun to metastasize. By that point, it is often too late for effective treatment.

TYPES OF OVARIAN CANCER

There are mainly two types of ovarian cancer—cystic and solid. *Cystic* means, simply, pertaining to a cyst—a mass filled with fluid.

Cystic ovarian cancer arises from the inner layer of the ovary. This kind of cyst can rupture and bleed. Such bleeding is often the first sign of ovarian cancer. But because it occurs when the tumor has grown big enough to rupture, such bleeding usually indicates an advanced stage. Sadly, cystic ovarian cancer sometimes occurs in teenagers.

A ruptured ovarian cyst presents an acute problem that requires immediate surgical intervention. The affected ovary must be removed. But because ovarian cancer often occurs at the same time in both ovaries, a biopsy must be performed on the second ovary as well. Ultrasound may also be used to observe whether the second ovary is enlarged. If it is, it also must be removed.

The second kind of ovarian cancer is called *adenocarcinoma*. It is the more common form of ovarian cancer, and it occurs later in life, most commonly after the age of fifty-five—though it can occur in woman as young as twenty.

Cancers that develop in women from teenagers to thirty are sometimes called *germ cell tumors*. These can be especially aggressive. Though they do not metastasize, they can be life threatening by virtue of their sheer size.

CAUSES AND PREVENTION OF OVARIAN CANCER

Risk factors for ovarian cancer may include genetic mutations (including BRCA1 and BRCA2), previous history of breast cancer, or family history of breast and ovarian cancer, or the use of fertility drugs may increase the risk. The more children a woman has, the lower her risk of ovarian cancer. Early age at first pregnancy and the use of some oral contraceptive pills have also been shown to have a protective effect.

Obviously, the removal of the ovaries isn't a procedure to take lightly. Where there's a strong family history of ovarian cancer, I will order genetic evaluation, and I'll provide counseling on the basis of

FIGURE 16

SEER INCIDENCE AND U.S. DEATH RATES,[+] 1975–2002

Ovary Cancer, by Age and Race

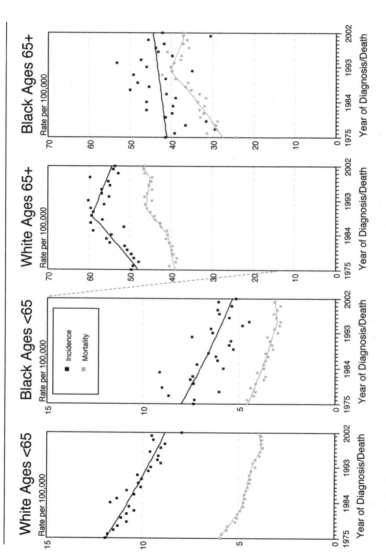

+ Source: SEER 9 areas and NCHS public use data file for the total US. Rates are age-adjusted to the 2000 US Std Population (19 age groups - Census P25-1103). Regression lines are calculated using the Joinpoint Regression Program Version 3.0, April 2005, National Cancer Institute.

Surveillance, Epidemiology, and End Results (SEER) Program (www.seer.cancer.gov) SEER*Stat Database: Incidence - SEER 9 Regs Public-Use, Nov 2004 Sub (1973-2002), National Cancer Institute, DCCPS, Surveillance Research Program, Cancer Statistics Branch, released April 2005, based on the November 2004 submission.

FIGURE 17

SEER INCIDENCE AND U.S. DEATH RATES, [†] 1975–2002

Ovary Cancer, by Age and Race

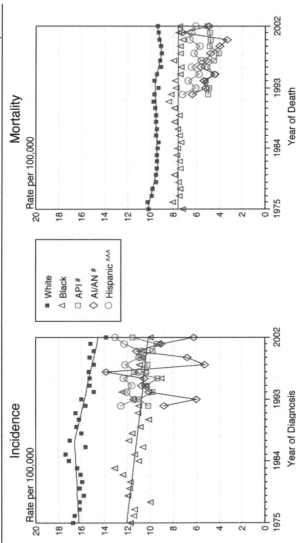

Joinpoint Analyses for 1975-2002 for Whites and Blacks
Rates for 1992-2002 for Asian/Pacific Islander, American Indian/Alaska Native and Hispanic

+ Source: Incidence data for whites and blacks is from the SEER 9 areas (San Francisco, Connecticut, Detroit, Hawaii, Iowa, New Mexico, Seattle, Utah, Atlanta). Incidence data for Asian/Pacific Islanders, American Indian/Alaska Natives and Hispanics is from the SEER 13 Areas (SEER 9 Areas, San Jose-Monterey, Los Angeles, Alaska Native Registry and Rural Georgia). Mortality data is from NCHS public use data file for the total US.
Rates are age-adjusted to the 2000 US Std Population (19 age groups - Census P25-1103).
Regression lines for whites and blacks are calculated using the Joinpoint Regression Program Version 3.0, April 2005, National Cancer Institute.

API = Asian/Pacific Islander. AI/AN = American Indian/Alaska Native.

^^^ Hispanic is not mutually exclusive from Whites, Blacks, Asian/Pacific Islanders, and American Indians/Alaska Natives. Incidence data for Hispanics excludes cases from Detroit, Hawaii, Alaska Native Registry and Rural Georgia. Mortality data for Hispanics excludes cases from Connecticut, Maine, Maryland, Minnesota, Oklahoma, New Hampshire, New York, North Dakota, and Vermont.

Surveillance, Epidemiology, and End Results (SEER) Program (www.seer.cancer.gov) SEER*Stat Database: Incidence - SEER 9 Regs Public-Use, Nov 2004 Sub (1973-2002), National Cancer Institute, DCCPS, Surveillance Research Program, Cancer Statistics Branch, released April 2005, based on the November 2004 submission.

it. Unless there are pressing reasons to perform surgery, I recommend regular pelvic exams and blood tests for tumor markers, the chemicals produced by the tumor, such as CA-125. Where there is a family history of ovarian cancer, I will also order ultrasound examinations every one or two years. The ultrasound will pick up enlarged ovaries. I will then check the ovary by means of a *laparoscopy* (a lighted instrument passed through the abdominal wall into the abdomen) or biopsy, or, if necessary, I will remove the ovary.

DIAGNOSING OVARIAN CANCER

Because of the large free space (peritoneal cavity) in the lining of the abdomen, ovarian cancer produces few early symptoms. A subtle but persistent discomfort may be the only symptom.

When a middle-aged patient complains of pelvic "fullness" or pain, too often this is dismissed as *pelvic inflammatory disease* (PID), a relatively benign condition. There are other conditions, too, that resemble the early stage of ovarian cancer and sometimes lead to misdiagnosis. These include *endometriosis* (abnormal tissue growth outside the uterus), and diseases of the colon.

Should you suffer from such symptoms, urge your doctor to explore *all* the possibilities. Too much is at stake here to neglect the possibility of a chance to diagnose ovarian cancer early.

Even symptoms of later stages of tumor growth can be mistaken for other diseases. These symptoms include cramping, nausea, or vomiting. If the tumor presses against the bladder, the patient will need to urinate more frequently. If the pressure is on the rectum, constipation or diarrhea can result.

For the doctor, this wide range of possibilities presents serious problems in diagnosis. Peptic ulcers, gallstones, or irritable bowel syndrome present similar symptoms.

Ask questions and insist on answers.

STAGING AND TREATMENT

If early diagnosis of ovarian cancer occurred more often, this section of the book could be more optimistic. When ovarian cancer is detected early and confined to one ovary, removal of that ovary results in better than 95 percent cure rates. Unfortunately, diagnosis of this cancer rarely is made early.

As with other cancers, researchers use a staging system to mark the progress of this disease—in this case, the system of the International Federation of Gynecology and Obstetrics (FIGO).

- Stage I: Tumor confined to the ovaries.
- Stage I A and B: No ascites (fluid accumulation); capsule intact.
- Stage I C: Capsule ruptured or ascites containing cancerous cells.
- Stage II: Tumor extension beyond ovaries in pelvis. May involve tubes or uterus.
- Stage II A, B, and C: Tumor may be present.
- Stage III: Peritoneal (in the membrane) implants outside pelvis.
- Stage III A, B, and C: Lymph nodes may be positive or negative.
- Stage IV: Extension outside abdomen—for example, in the chest—with proven tumor; metastases inside liver (blood-borne).

As I've said, approximately 5 percent of ovarian cancers are genetic—that is, they run in families. Women who have had mothers, grandmothers, or aunts stricken with the disease should consider prophylactic (preventive) removal of the ovaries. Even so drastic a treatment, however, isn't always effective. In some cases, *primary peritoneal carcinomatosis*—that is, the spread of the cancer to the peritoneum, or lining of the abdominal cavity—develops after the ovaries have been surgically removed.

Again, because surgical removal is so drastic a procedure, and because it is not a guarantee against ovarian cancer, some women who feel at risk because of family history may prefer annual pelvic exams with vaginal ultrasound and measurements of CA-125.

Often, the cruelest fact about cancer is that it requires one to live with uncertainty. *Am I cured or not? Will this procedure repay the suffering it may cost by adding years to my life? If I refuse this treatment, am I failing to fight as hard as I should?* These are difficult, even terrible questions. But many women have found ways to live with them and you can, too. My own view is that you'll do better if you talk about your fears with your doctor, and with others, too—spouse or other loved ones, minister, social worker. If you're in a support group, all the better. There you can share your fears with others who have wrestled with them.

Often, the cruelest fact about cancer is that it requires one to live with uncertainty.

Ovarian cancer is especially cruel because most women are in stage III when first diagnosed. At that stage, surgery is the only real option. The surgeon will attempt to remove as much of the tumor as possible without doing injury to other organs. This usually means removal of both tubes, ovaries, and uterus with *omentum,* a fatty apron hanging from the colon. The surgeon will also biopsy any peritoneal implants or lymph nodes in the groin and within the abdominal cavity. When no implants are noted, the surgeon will wash the abdominal cavity with a solution that can be "spun down" and checked under a microscope for tumor cells.

You'll do better if you talk about your fears.

If surgery reveals that the cancer has spread beyond the ovaries, causing ascites, or liquid accumulation, the surgeon may install a chemotherapeutic agent or administer chemotherapy after the surgery has been completed. Certainly, a stage III or stage IV ovarian cancer will require such follow-up treatment. The usual chemical agents are either cisplatin or carboplatin. Some doctors will also order external radiation of the abdomen as part of the follow-up treatment.

Elderly patients can present special problems. Sometimes they must receive chemotherapy before surgery, in the hope that the treatment will make the tumor more operable. Often the elderly must be given extra fluids and nutritional support to build them up for the surgery.

Regardless of the age of the patient, it's the surgeon's job to remove as much tumor as is feasible—we call this *debulking*. Where the bowels are involved in the cancer, sections must be removed (resected). Tumor deposits on the lining (peritoneum) of the abdominal wall must also be removed, along with any lymph nodes that are involved.

Monitoring the status of ovarian cancer after treatment is difficult but necessary. Your doctor may order a *second-look operation,* or laparoscopy. Tumor markers that are helpful in the case of other cancers may be less effective here.

Such follow-up operations are appropriate only for patients strong enough to tolerate them. In some cases, these operations may require the removal of new tumors, and this can mean further resectioning of the bowels. In other cases, the surgeon may simply repeat his or her earlier procedure of biopsy, washings, and so forth. Your doctor may decide after the second-look operation that further chemotherapy is warranted.

A common cause of death in the case of ovarian cancer is bowel obstruction. In some cases, the doctor may order surgery involving further resectioning of the bowel and removal of the obstruction. Such surgery may make the patient more comfortable, but it will not improve her overall condition. Further, it is fraught with danger because the tumor is so extensive. Removing it, along with a section of the colon, involves high risk of leakage of the bowel and a resulting peritonitis infection.

Because surgery in this case is difficult and dangerous, the doctor may instead make the patient more comfortable by having a tube placed in the stomach to decompress the obstructed bowel and to feed the patient intravenously. I think that's usually the better choice.

PROGNOSIS FOR OVARIAN CANCER

Because ovarian cancer is usually quite advanced by the time diagnosis is made, the outcome is often poor. The five-year survival rate for 1995–2001 for all stages was 44.67 percent. If, however, diagnosis is made early in the disease, five-year survival rates can reach 94 percent.

To sum up, ovarian cancer is the fourth leading cause of cancer deaths among women. There are few early symptoms. As the disease progresses, nonspecific symptoms like frequency of urination, "fullness," and nausea occur. A strong family history with the disease should prompt a workup for ovarian cancer. Such a workup should include pelvic exam, vaginal ultrasound, and CA-125. Prophylactic (preventive) removal of the ovaries should also be considered for patients with strong family history.

The essence of treatment of ovarian cancer is surgical removal of as much tumor as possible with accurate staging followed by chemotherapy if tumor is left behind.

In African-American women, it is important to include the consideration of ovarian cancer in any patient with pelvic symptoms. Because PID (pelvic inflammatory disease) is considered common to African-American women, too often they are so diagnosed when they have pelvic pain.

IN A NUTSHELL

Incidence:
Ovarian cancer accounts for approximately 4 percent of all women's cancers and is the fourth leading cause of cancer-related death among women in the United States. The incidence rate for ovarian cancer has been slowly declining since the early 1990s. Ovarian cancer has the highest mortality of all

cancers of the female reproductive system, which reflects, in part, a lack of early symptoms and proven ovarian cancer screening tests. Thus, ovarian cancer is often diagnosed at an advanced stage, after the cancer has spread beyond the ovary. White women have higher incidence and mortality rates than other racial and ethnic groups. It is estimated that approximately $2.2 billion is spent in the United States each year on treatment of ovarian cancer.

Risk Factors:
Genetic mutations, previous history of breast cancer, or family history of breast and ovarian cancer all may increase risk. The use of fertility drugs may also be a risk factor.

Prevention:
Bilateral *oophorectomy* (removal of ovaries) to be considered if there is strong family history—but only within the framework described in this chapter.

Diagnosis:
- Be alert to nonspecific pressure symptoms, nausea, vomiting, abdominal and pelvic pain, especially if you have a familial history of ovarian cancer.
- Your doctor will do a pelvic exam, with the purpose of detecting pelvic mass. He may also employ vaginal ultrasound, CA-125, laparoscopy and biopsy, or a pelvic exploration aided by surgery.

Treatment:
- Surgical removal of ovaries for prophylaxis (prevention)
- Removal of ovaries, tubes, and uturus; debulk and stage; chemotherapy.

Prognosis:
The five-year survival rate for all stages is only 35–38 percent. If, however, diagnosis is made early in the disease, five-year survival rates can reach 90–98 percent.

THIRTEEN

Bladder Cancer

L OUISE SULLIVAN HAD BEEN reading quietly. When her husband, Marvin, heard her cry out from the bathroom, he rushed to her side. He could see she was frightened. At first, she wouldn't speak. Then she said, quietly because she was trying so hard to control herself, "Honey, I need to see the doctor. There was blood in my urine." Louise had been complaining for a week of an uncomfortable feeling in her lower abdomen, and now she recognized the blood as the red-light warning signal that it was.

That's how it happened that Louise got diagnosed early and treated effectively. Since she was diagnosed and treated, she comes in for checkups regularly. That's why now, some three years later, she's doing so well.

INCIDENCE AND MORTALITY

During 2005, according to National Cancer Institute estimates, new cases of bladder cancer will amount to, in men, 38,000 new cases and in women, 15,000 new cases. Among men bladder cancer is the fourth most common type of cancer, and among women the eighth most common. The incidence rate and the mortality rates are lower for African Americans than for whites.

RISK FACTORS

Smokers have nearly five times more chance of developing bladder cancer than nonsmokers. By quitting smoking, you decrease the risk. Workplace exposure to carcinogens accounts for about one in four cases. Arylamines are a group of chemicals most responsible. Dye workers, rubber workers, aluminum workers, leather workers, truck drivers, and pesticide applicators are at the highest risk. Women who received radiation treatment for cervical cancer have an increased risk of developing transitional cell bladder cancer. A chronic (long-term) bladder infection or irritation may lead to the development of squamous bladder cancer, but this cancer is slow in developing.

SYMPTOMS

The usual presenting symptom—that is, the primary symptom that most commonly brings the patient to the doctor's office—is *hematuria*, or blood in the urine. Later, the patient will experience *dysuria* (painful urination), and a more frequent than normal need to urinate.

The ureters (tubes carrying urine from kidney to bladder) may also become obstructed. If that happens, it will result in *hydronephrosis* (water- or urine-logged kidneys) and *uremia* (backup of urine waste products in the blood). These two conditions will produce symptoms of vomiting, insomnia, and muscular weakness.

DIAGNOSIS

When your doctor sees symptoms of bladder cancer, he will probably refer you to a urologist. The urologist will do a *cystoscopy* (an observation of the bladder by means of a lighted instrument placed

FIGURE 18

SEER INCIDENCE, DELAY-ADJUSTED INCIDENCE AND U.S. DEATH RATES, [†] 1975–2002

Urinary Bladder Cancer, by Race and Sex

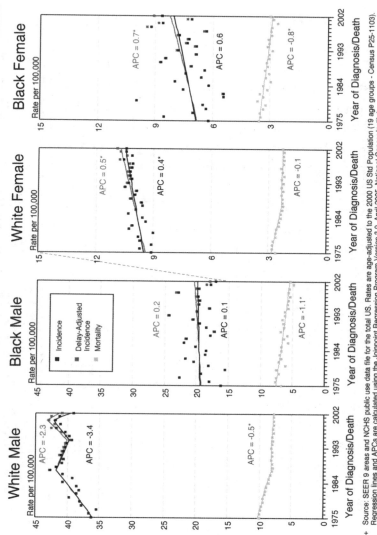

+ Source: SEER 9 areas and NCHS public use data file for the total US. Rates are age-adjusted to the 2000 US Std Population (19 age groups - Census P25-1103).
  Regression lines and APCs are calculated using the Joinpoint Regression Program Version 3.0, April 2005, National Cancer Institute.
  The APC is the Annual Percent Change for the regression line segments. The APC shown on the graph is for the most recent trend.
* The APC is significantly different from zero (p < 0.05).

Surveillance, Epidemiology, and End Results (SEER) Program (www.seer.cancer.gov) SEER*Stat Database: Incidence - SEER 9 Regs Public-Use, Nov 2004 Sub (1973-2002), National Cancer Institute, DCCPS, Surveillance Research Program, Cancer Statistics Branch, released April 2005, based on the November 2004 submission.

FIGURE 19

SEER INCIDENCE AND U.S. DEATH RATES,[+] 1975–2002

Urinary Bladder Cancer, Both Sexes

Joinpoint Analyses for 1975-2002 for Whites and Blacks
Rates for 1992-2002 for Asian/Pacific Islander, American Indian/Alaska Native and Hispanic

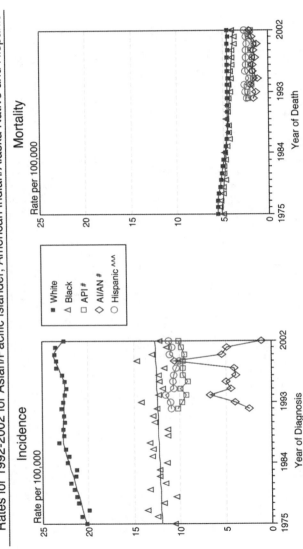
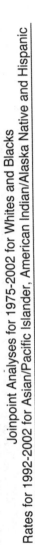

+ Source: Incidence data for whites and blacks is from the SEER 9 areas (San Francisco, Connecticut, Detroit, Hawaii, Iowa, New Mexico, Seattle, Utah, Atlanta).
Incidence data for Asian/Pacific Islanders, American Indian/Alaska Natives and Hispanics is from the SEER 13 Areas (SEER 9 Areas, San Jose-Monterey, Los Angeles,
Alaska Native Registry and Rural Georgia). Mortality data is from NCHS public use data file for the total US.
Rates are age-adjusted to the 2000 US Std Population (19 age groups - Census P25-1103).
Regression lines for whites and blacks are calculated using the Joinpoint Regression Program Version 3.0, April 2005, National Cancer Institute.
API = Asian/Pacific Islander. AI/AN = American Indian/Alaska Native.
^^^ Hispanic is not mutually exclusive from Whites, Blacks, Asian/Pacific Islanders, and American Indians/Alaska Natives. Incidence data for Hispanics excludes
cases from Detroit, Hawaii, Alaska Native Registry and Rural Georgia. Mortality data for Hispanics excludes cases from Connecticut, Maine, Maryland, Minnesota,
Oklahoma, New Hampshire, New York, North Dakota, and Vermont.

Surveillance, Epidemiology, and End Results (SEER) Program (www.seer.cancer.gov) SEER*Stat Database: Incidence - SEER 9 Regs Public-Use,
Nov 2004 Sub (1973-2002), National Cancer Institute, DCCPS, Surveillance Research Program, Cancer Statistics Branch, released April 2005,
based on the November 2004 submission.

in the bladder. During the process, he will do a biopsy, from which a specific diagnosis can be made.

An x-ray of the kidney, called IVP (*intravenous pyelogram*), is done to assess the status of the kidneys. CT scanning can be used to assist in staging. And staging will depend on the depth of penetration into the wall of the bladder and the local and distal (that is, how far away from the point of origin) spread of the tumor.

These are the main features of each stage of the disease:

- Stage 0: Confined to mucosa or on the surface of the inner lining of the bladder.
- Stage I: Cancer cells are found deep in the inner lining of the bladder but have not spread to the muscle of the bladder.
- Stage II: The cancer cells have spread to the muscle of the bladder.
- Stage III: The cancer cells have spread through the muscular wall of the bladder to the layer of tissue surrounding the bladder. The cancer cells may have spread to the prostate (in men) or to the uterus or vagina (in women).
- Stage IV: The cancer extends to the wall of the abdomen or to the wall of the pelvis. The cancer cells may have spread to lymph nodes and other parts of the body far away from the bladder, such as the lungs.

TREATMENT

Because bleeding is an early symptom, most bladder tumors are caught early. Superficial tumors (stages 0 and I) can be removed surgically or by means of electric current (*fulguration*) through the urethra (the tube from the bladder used for urinating).

Chemotherapeutic agents or immunotherapy can be introduced into the bladder.

Where the tumor has penetrated deeply into the muscular wall of the bladder, more definitive surgery is required. The preferred treatment is *radical cystectomy* (removal of the bladder). In such cases, the surgeon will make a new bladder to do the work of the old.

PROGNOSIS

For superficial lesions, prognosis is good. Where the condition is neglected and the tumor allowed to spread, prognosis is poor.

IN A NUTSHELL

Incidence:
Each year an estimated 53,000 new cases of cancer of the bladder occur in Americans, and each year about 13,180 Americans will die of it.

Risk Factors:
Smokers have nearly five times more chance of developing bladder cancer than nonsmokers. By quitting smoking, you decrease the risk. Workplace exposure to carcinogens accounts for about one in four cases. Arylamines are a group of chemicals most responsible. Dye workers, rubber workers, aluminum workers, leather workers, truck drivers, and pesticide applicators are at the highest risk. Women who received radiation treatment for cervical cancer have an increased risk of developing transitional cell bladder cancer. A chronic (long-term) bladder infection or irritation may lead to the development of squamous bladder cancer, but this cancer is slow in developing.

Prevention:
Stop smoking, or don't start.

Diagnosis:
Cancer of the bladder presents with early hematuria, and therefore can usually be diagnosed and treated early, when the prognosis is good.

Treatment:
- Stages 0 and I: Local/fulguration
- Stages II and III: Cystectomy
- Stage IV: X-ray and chemotherapy.

Prognosis
- Stages 0 and I: Good
- Stage II: Fair
- Stage III: Guarded
- Stage IV: Poor.

FOURTEEN

Kidney Cancer

MARVIN HAD BEEN A SMOKER for a long time, and a lucky one at that. He exercised, ate well, took care of himself. "Smoking is my only vice," he liked to say. And he secretly thought he was the exception that maybe proved the rule—he'd never suffered severely from breathing problems, and his heart was all right.

Then, out of the blue, trouble struck. Marvin began to suffer a pain in his right groin, something like a cramp that became more and more permanent. He talked with friends who suggested that the cause might be a kidney stone. And he waited a little longer.

It was only when he saw blood in his urine that he finally visited his doctor. "Funny thing is," Marvin told him, "I felt better after passing the clot. But, still, there was something about that blood in my urine that made me pay attention."

KIDNEY CANCER AND AFRICAN AMERICANS

About 32,000 new cases of kidney cancer are diagnosed each year. Of these 12,600 will die, approximately one-fourth of these African Americans.

SYMPTOMS

Among the most common symptoms of kidney cancer are:

- A tumor in the side or the abdomen
- Pain in the side that does not go away
- Blood in the urine (hematuria)
- Fever
- Weight loss
- Fatigue.

The most pronounced symptoms of kidney cancer appear in the late stages of the disease and in only half the cases. Bleeding is caused when the tumor erodes into the tube that drains urine from the kidney. The pain is caused by the stretching of the kidney itself under pressure of the tumor.

Passing of blood clots will cause cramps that mimic kidney stones. Fever may also occur, and may mistakenly suggest a kidney infection. The cause of the fever isn't certain, but it may be due to the death (*necrosis*) of tumor cells or to actual infection that results when the tumor blocks the kidney's draining system.

DIAGNOSIS

Fortunately, kidney cancer is usually diagnosed early, before major symptoms occur, because nonspecific abdominal symptoms routinely result in a CT scan being done.

SEER INCIDENCE AND U.S. DEATH RATES, [†] 1975–2002
Kidney and Renal Pelvis Cancer, Both Sexes

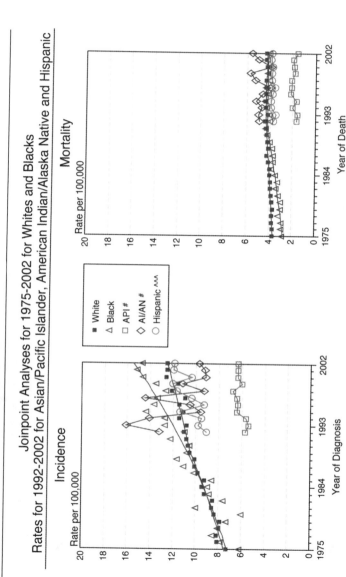

Joinpoint Analyses for 1975-2002 for Whites and Blacks
Rates for 1992-2002 for Asian/Pacific Islander, American Indian/Alaska Native and Hispanic

[†] Source: Incidence data for whites and blacks is from the SEER 9 areas (San Francisco, Connecticut, Detroit, Hawaii, Iowa, New Mexico, Seattle, Utah, Atlanta). Incidence data for Asian/Pacific Islanders, American Indian/Alaska Natives and Hispanics is from the SEER 13 Areas (SEER 9 Areas, San Jose-Monterey, Los Angeles, Alaska Native Registry and Rural Georgia). Mortality data is from NCHS public use data file for the total US. Rates are age-adjusted to the 2000 US Std Population (19 age groups - Census P25-1103). Regression lines for whites and blacks are calculated using the Joinpoint Regression Program Version 3.0, April 2005, National Cancer Institute.
API = Asian/Pacific Islander. AI/AN = American Indian/Alaska Native.
^^^ Hispanic is not mutually exclusive from Whites, Blacks, Asian/Pacific Islanders, and American Indians/Alaska Natives. Incidence data for Hispanics excludes cases from Detroit, Hawaii, Alaska Native Registry and Rural Georgia. Mortality data for Hispanics excludes cases from Connecticut, Maine, Maryland, Minnesota, Oklahoma, New Hampshire, New York, North Dakota, and Vermont.

Surveillance, Epidemiology, and End Results (SEER) Program (www.seer.cancer.gov) SEER*Stat Database: Incidence - SEER 9 Regs Public-Use, Nov 2004 Sub (1973-2002), National Cancer Institute, DCCPS, Surveillance Research Program, Cancer Statistics Branch, released April 2005, based on the November 2004 submission.

Occasionally, an *angiogram* (an x-ray of the blood vessels high-lighted by injected dye) or intravenous phelogram (IVP) is used to determine if a tumor has invaded the abdominal area. But because the CT scan provides greater clarity, it is the preferred method.

TREATMENT

When kidney cancer is diagnosed, removal of the kidney, adrenal gland, and lymph nodes (*radical nephrectomy*) is the most common treatment of choice. Metastases, if any have occurred, may diminish after the primary tumor has been removed. As in the case of colon cancer, isolated metastases—in the lung or the liver, for example—can be removed with good results.

Chemotherapy has shown limited use against kidney cancer.

PROGNOSIS

Like other cancers, kidney cancer is staged from I to IV. Stage I is an early stage with cells found only in the kidney. In stage IV, the cancer has spread beyond the tissue surrounding the kidney, to other parts of the body, or is found in more than one nearby lymph node.

Kidney cancer is one of those uncommon cancers that is usually caught early. Of course, the later it is diagnosed, the poorer the prognosis. Overall, about one patient in three dies of this disease.

IN A NUTSHELL

Incidence:

Some 32,000 cases of kidney cancer are estimated each year. Of these, some 12,000 will die, accounting for 2 percent of all cancer deaths. Some 3,700 African Americans are diagnosed with it each year, and each year, some 1,100 African Americans die of it.

Cause:
Unknown but related to smoking

Prevention:
Stop smoking, or don't start.

Diagnosis:
Be alert to flank pain, cramps, blood in urine, and palpable tumor mass.

Your physician will:
- Take your medical history, checking for tumor mass
- Do a CT scan, sometimes an angiogram as well.

Treatment:
Radical removal of kidney.

Prognosis:
Good if early (70 percent); poor if late.

FIFTEEN

Cancer of the Esophagus

DARRELL'S CASE

AS HE AND HIS WIFE AND FRIENDS came to the table, Darrell Holmes took pleasure in the moment. Why not? His wife, Alice, now seated across from him, wore her special glow, and they were sharing this meal with their friends, Arnold and Belle. The room was soft with candlelight and laughter. As to the food, it was just what the doctor ordered, Darrell said when Alice brought it to the table—steak, potatoes fried as only Alice knew how to fry them, asparagus, and plenty of good red wine. "Fit for a king, fit for a king," Darrell thought. And why not? He'd struggled to pay his way through college and law school, and now, at forty, he was enjoying the fruits.

But when Darrell swallowed the first bit of steak, he knew there was something bitter in the fruit. The bite felt as if it was stuck in his chest and wouldn't pass into his stomach. It was accompanied by a burning pain. Darrell drank a few sips of water, and it gave him some relief. But a moment later, when he tried again to swallow a piece of meat, the same thing happened.

Darrell excused himself to take some over-the-counter antacid medicine and felt better. But when the meal was over, he'd left most of his steak on the plate. "Don't know what it is," he told Alice and their friends. "Maybe my body's telling me to become a vegetarian."

Darrell didn't believe that, but, in the next few months, his diet did change. He wanted soft things, which were also high in fats. No more steaks or roasts or chops for him. At first, the soft diet went down better. But gradually Darrell lost all desire to eat. He was losing weight, and Alice was worried. Still, Darrell refused to see a doctor.

What finally turned him around was that he could no longer swallow his saliva. It built up, causing him to cough and sometimes choke. It felt as if his lungs were being affected by this buildup of body liquids he couldn't get rid of. He wasn't breathing well, and he coughed a lot. That's when he went to the doctor.

ESOPHAGEAL CANCER AND BLACKS

The incidence of esophageal cancer in the United States is low (about 1 percent of all cancers), but it is rising, in part because of rising obesity rates. The estimated number of new cases in 2005, according to the American Cancer Society, is 14,520, and the estimated number of deaths is 13,570.

As you can see, this cancer is especially lethal. African American men are one to three times as likely as whites to have cancer of the esophagus, African-American women almost twice as likely. White males have five-year-survival rate of 16.1 and white females, 16.4. But in African Americans these numbers are 8.6 and 11.6.

Esophogeal cancer is relatively rare in the United States. But it is so deadly that incidence and mortality rates are not far apart. Men are more likely than women to have this form of cancer. While the incidence rate for African Americans has dropped sharply, they are still higher than the incidence rate for whites, at approximately 10/100,000 against 8/100,000. While the mortality rate for African

SEER INCIDENCE, DELAY-ADJUSTED INCIDENCE AND U.S. DEATH RATES,[†] 1975–2002

Esophagus Cancer, by Race and Sex

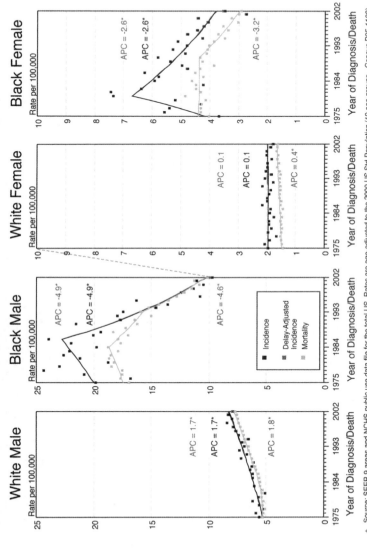

Source: SEER 9 areas and NCHS public use data file for the total US. Rates are age-adjusted to the 2000 US Std Population (19 age groups - Census P25-1103). Regression lines and APCs are calculated using the Joinpoint Regression Program Version 3.0, April 2005, National Cancer Institute.
The APC is the Annual Percent Change for the regression line segments. The APC shown on the graph is for the most recent trend.
* The APC is significantly different from zero (p < 0.05).

Surveillance, Epidemiology, and End Results (SEER) Program (www.seer.cancer.gov) SEER*Stat Database: Incidence - SEER 9 Regs Public-Use, Nov 2004 Sub (1973-2002), National Cancer Institute, DCCPS, Surveillance Research Program, Cancer Statistics Branch, released April 2005, based on the November 2004 submission.

FIGURE 22

SEER INCIDENCE AND U.S. DEATH RATES,[†] 1975–2002

Esophagus Cancer, Both Sexes

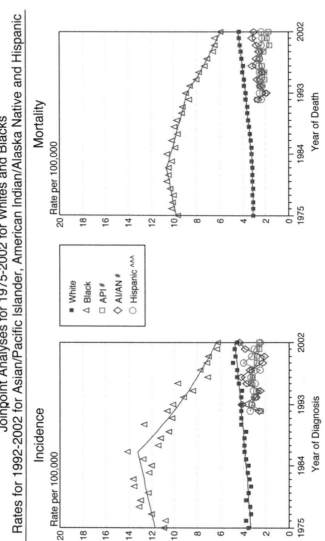

Joinpoint Analyses for 1975-2002 for Whites and Blacks
Rates for 1992-2002 for Asian/Pacific Islander, American Indian/Alaska Native and Hispanic

† Source: Incidence data for whites and blacks is from the SEER 9 areas (San Francisco, Connecticut, Detroit, Hawaii, Iowa, New Mexico, Seattle, Utah, Atlanta).
Incidence data for Asian/Pacific Islanders, American Indian/Alaska Natives and Hispanics is from the SEER 13 Areas (SEER 9 Areas, San Jose-Monterey, Los Angeles,
Alaska Native Registry and Rural Georgia). Mortality data is from NCHS public use data file for the total US.
Rates are age-adjusted to the 2000 US Std Population (19 age groups - Census P25-1103).
Regression lines for whites and blacks are calculated using the Joinpoint Regression Program Version 3.0, April 2005, National Cancer Institute.
API = Asian/Pacific Islander. AI/AN = American Indian/Alaska Native.
^^^ Hispanic is not mutually exclusive from Whites, Blacks, Asian/Pacific Islanders, and American Indians/Alaska Natives. Incidence data for Hispanics excludes
cases from Detroit, Hawaii, Alaska Native Registry and Rural Georgia. Mortality data for Hispanics excludes cases from Connecticut, Maine, Maryland, Minnesota,
Oklahoma, New Hampshire, New York, North Dakota, and Vermont.

Surveillance, Epidemiology, and End Results (SEER) Program (www.seer.cancer.gov) SEER*Stat Database: Incidence - SEER 9 Regs Public-Use,
Nov 2004 Sub (1973-2002), National Cancer Institute, DCCPS, Surveillance Research Program, Cancer Statistics Branch, released April 2005,

Americans has also dropped, it is still higher for African Americans than for whites. Mortality rates for African Americans have also dropped, but, again, they are higher in African Americans.

CAUSES

Smoking and alcohol are the primary risk factors of esophageal cancer. Age, sex (it is more common in males) and long-term irritation are also risk factors.

PREVENTION

Because the primary risk factors are fairly well documented, the preventive measures are clear: don't smoke and don't drink.

ANATOMY OF THE ESOPHAGUS

Before we can say more about this aggressive disease, we must tell you something about the esophagus itself. The esophagus is a thin tube made up primarily of muscle. Food passes through the esophagus from the pharynx into the stomach. This means that the esophagus also passes through the chest.

Food is carried through the esophagus down into the stomach as a result of the tube's contraction. Gravity plays only a limited role in the act of swallowing.

The esophagus is divided into three segments, all deeply embedded in the body. The first is the cervical esophagus (located in the neck), then the thoracic esophagus (located in the chest), and lastly the short abdominal esophagus (located in the abdomen below the diaphragm).

Because the esophagus passes through three different compartments, esophageal cancer presents special problems to the surgeon in that the surgical approach can be through the chest, neck, or abdomen, depending on which part of the esophagus is affected.

FIGURE 23

ANATOMY OF ESOPHAGUS, STOMACH, SMALL INTESTINE

Sometimes, if the disease involves the entire length of the esophagus, the surgeon must make three separate incisions to reach the three different segments.

The wall of the esophagus comprises three thin layers of tissue. The muscle layer is the primary working part, providing the essential function of peristalsis (muscle contractions that propel food in a downward direction). Lining the inside of the esophagus is a layer of specialized tissue that protects the wall against ingested bacteria; environmental contaminants; and digestive juices, including saliva. Finally, the outside coat encases the esophagus and isolates it from such surrounding structures as the aorta, bronchus, and trachea.

This outer membrane is fragile and poorly developed. Diseases of the esophagus penetrate it easily to invade surrounding structures. Diseases of the esophagus usually begin either in the muscular layer or the inside lining. Cancer itself usually starts from the innermost layer.

PHYSIOLOGY OF THE ESOPHAGUS

The esophagus carries food to the stomach. As the esophagus empties food into the acid-filled stomach, a small amount of that liquid acid may leak back up into the esophagus. If that happens often or over a prolonged time, the acid can injure the esophagus. This *reflux* (backup) of gastric acid sometimes causes pain. But it can also go undetected and untreated for a long time. When that happens, significant damage, sometimes including cancer, can occur.

SYMPTOMS

You know something about the symptoms of esophogeal cancer already from Darrell's case. Symptoms include:

- Difficulty swallowing
- A lump and/or pain in the throat
- Loss of appetite and weight loss
- Fatigue
- Weakness
- Indigestion and heartburn
- Hoarseness or chronic cough
- Coughing up blood.

Because these symptoms can be mistaken for symptoms of other diseases, the doctor must listen with particular care to the patient's account of the history of the disease and present complaints. Doctors must also make special efforts to get beyond language and cultural barriers. Diagnosis will depend on the doctor's own communication and listening skills.

A word or two more is necessary about the problems created by the patient's difficulty in swallowing saliva. Saliva builds up because the esophagus is blocked by the cancerous mass. The patient must spit constantly. But even spitting can't relieve the constant buildup. Some saliva, or liquid taken by mouth, may spill over into the lungs. This will result in pneumonia, which antiobiotics can only temporarily control.

If the tumor continues to grow, it will also disable muscles of the esophagus. When the muscles are no longer able to contract, food and saliva will accumulate so that the esophagus itself balloons out.

As the tumor grows, it will break through the wall of the esophagus, and where it breaks through, bleeding occurs. The cancer can also invade the blood vessels, causing even more rapid blood loss.

For these reasons, blood in the stool, identified by a simple test, is often an early warning of esophageal cancer. Though the blood can have other causes, it at least shows that the source of the problem is limited to the gastrointestinal (digestive) tract.

Pain is rarely an early symptom of esophageal cancer. Heartburn may occur, though it isn't a result of the cancer so much as of the acid backup from stomach to esophagus that causes cancer.

Weakness, tiredness, severe weight loss, and chronic fatigue are common symptoms, but they're nonspecific—that is, they are signs of many illnesses.

DIAGNOSIS

The preferred method for diagnosing esophageal cancer is called endoscopy or EGD (endoscopic gastroduodenoscopy). The endoscope is a long, thin, flexible tube that contains optical fibers to illuminate the inside of the esophagus and stomach. Biopsies are obtained through the use of flexible instruments inserted down the tube.

Endoscopy is a quick outpatient procedure that requires no more than ten to twenty minutes. With the help of sedatives and drugs that induce amnesia, the experience is painless and immediately forgotten. To prevent vomiting, patients should not eat for at least eight hours before the procedure.

Don't be shocked when, at the start of the procedure, the doctor or technician asks you to wear a mouth guard. That is necessary to prevent you from involuntarily biting and damaging the scope while under sedation.

A barium esophagram is a second diagnostic method that, though less used, is an acceptable alternative to, and has certain advantages over, endoscopy. In emergency cases a barium esophagram is quicker because the patient need not empty his or her stomach. It is also painless and requires no sedation.

The barium esophogram starts with the patient drinking a liquid containing barium. While the patient is lying on a table, the radiologist views the esophagus with the help of fluoroscopy (continuous x-ray). Where the radiologist observes abrupt changes in the flow of barium, he or she will take a picture. Cancers of the esophagus have a characteristic appearance and are easily diagnosed by the radiologist though, in some cases, a tissue diagnosis is also necessary, and that will require an EGD.

When esophageal cancer has been diagnosed, further studies are done to determine the spread of the disease.

CT scans can identify tumors that are 1 cm or more long. But CT scans show *all* tumors, including benign ones.

Finally, a new special endoscope with a built-in ultrasonic probe is available in some medical centers. Sound waves detail all layers of the esophageal wall and allow the doctor to determine the depth of wall penetrations, an observation necessary to staging the cancer.

TREATMENT

Treatment of esophageal cancer involves a combination of surgery, chemotherapy, radiation and laser therapy. As with most cancers, early diagnosis means a better chance of survival. It also means a better chance of effective surgery. But in general, the prognosis for this disease is poor.

Surgery

Surgery—the preferred treatment for stage I cancers—involves removal of the portion of the esophagus that contains the cancer. But though visible and palpable tumors can be removed in this way, cancer also spreads microscopically, in groups of cells too small to be seen or felt by the surgeon. For that reason, the surgeon will generally remove an additional 5 cm of the esophagus beyond the extent of the tumor. By removing this apparently healthy margin, the surgeon stands a better chance of removing the cancer completely.

Another approach is to remove the esophagus completely, replacing it with a section of the stomach. This approach is still under debate and awaits future clinical trials for resolution.

Surgery is a necessary part of the treatment, but it presents many difficulties. For one, the surgery itself is difficult. We have already spoken of the necessity, in some cases, of working in three separate body compartments—the neck, chest, and abdomen—through three separate incisions.

The surgeon is also challenged by the complex job of freeing up the stomach, fashioning it into a tube to replace the esophagus, then, through the chest, removing the diseased organ itself. If the cancer is in the upper segment of the esophagus, or if the entire esophagus is removed, the stomach must be made to reach to the neck, where it is reconnected to the cervical portion of the esophagus or to the pharynx. This requires an additional incision in the neck.

Even in this simplified version, it is obvious that the operation is challenging to the surgeon and very hard on the patient as well.

Until quite recently, 20 percent of the patients died following surgery, of malnutrition, of poor lungs weakened by years of smoking, or of the relatively crude techniques of reconstruction then available.

The use of the stomach itself as the material with which to refashion the esophagus has improved matters, but the surgical attachment of stomach to remaining esophagus or pharynx is fragile. Dangers of leakage and subsequent infection are very real.

Radiation

Surgery alone is the preferred treatment for stage I cancers—those limited to the inner lining. But most patients present to the doctor only when they are in advanced stages of the disease. In such cases, surgery alone can relieve symptoms and prevent the local complications that result from growth of the mass. But in such cases, surgery rarely cures. And the risks from surgery, together with poor long-term survival rates, make other kinds of treatment more attractive.

Radiation can be used to remove or shrink cancerous masses of the esophagus. Today, computers allow precise targeting and precise doses of radiation. The result is that normal tissues are spared the harmful effects of the radiation.

The upshot is that patients in advanced stages of esophageal cancer can be treated with radiation. The results, though far from perfect, are as good as those obtained by surgery for patients with advanced stages of esophageal cancer. In those cases where the right balance between just enough and too much radiation can be achieved, the pain of the cancer can be eased and its growth slowed. But advanced esophageal cancer always leads to death.

Chemotherapy

Used alone, current chemotherapy has little to offer. What it *does* offer is to boost the therapeutic effects of radiation and therefore allow smaller doses of radiation to be used. The combination of chemotherapy and radiation, along with the many difficulties posed by the surgery itself, has raised the question of whether surgery is needed at all in the treatment of esophageal cancer.

DARRELL TODAY

Darrell was treated with combination therapy, and he is doing moderately well six months later. He's had to change a lot of habits. Not only has he given up smoking and alcohol, but he's on a new diet, low in fat, high in fresh fruits and vegetables. He's also begun to exercise—at first, by walking around the block. Now he's joined a gym where he's doing some light but regular exercise.

We asked Darrell how he felt about his new life. "I'm a much humbler man," he said. "I thought I was immortal. Funny thing is, I kind of like this new feeling of vulnerability. I think I've grown kinder. But, you see, it's also that I don't know how much time I've got. Actually, when I think about it, I never *did* know. But now it's real, immediate. I don't know how to say it, but it's changed the way I look at things. My wife's beauty, a new leaf, a baby in a stroller I see in the street—I can't tell you how bright those things shine out at me now."

IN A NUTSHELL

Incidence:
Incidence rates are, for whites, 4.6/100,000; and for blacks, 6.21/100,000. There is also a gap in death rates: white, 4.3/100,000; black 5.9/100,000.

Cause:
Smoking, alcohol.

Prevention:
Don't smoke, and don't drink.

Diagnosis:
Be alert to:
- difficulty swallowing
- a lump in the throat
- loss of appetite and weight loss
- fatigue.

- weakness

  Your doctor will use endoscopy (with or without ultrasound probe) or barium esophogram.

Treatment:
- Stage I: surgery
- Advanced stages: radiation and chemotherapy, often in combination.

Prognosis:

Survival rates are 13 percent for whites, 9 percent for blacks.

SIXTEEN

Stomach Cancer

JANICE'S CASE

JANICE SIMMONS WAS THE ENVY of her friends. Still healthy and vigorous at sixty-six, Janice spent time with her grandchildren, and worked six hours a week at the church office. She saw her physician, Dr. Ngnale, regularly, and that was one of the many ways she made her doctor happy. His job was simply to keep her healthy.

Dr. Ngnale made sure Janice got the routine physical exams and that, once a year, she had:

- A Pap smear
- A mammogram
- A hemoccult test (a test to check for blood in the stool)
- A cholesterol and blood sugar test.

Three years ago, she had a sigmoidoscopic exam checking for polyps in her colon. She had none, and wouldn't need another test for several more years.

Janice's only real medical problem was hypertension (high blood pressure). Indeed, it was her fear of stroke that kept her going so regularly to Dr. Ngnale. Her mother had died ten years ago after complications from a sudden, massive stroke. Janice remembered vividly the agony of seeing her mother unable to speak or walk, and the terrible upheavals the whole family had gone through trying to decide between nursing-home care and full-time home care.

Dr. Ngnale knew of Janice's concern and he shared it. He made sure she took an aspirin each night along with the hormone pill Premarin®. He had also been encouraging her for years to change her diet but hadn't had much luck winning her over. Still, all in all, Janice Simmons was healthy, and Dr. Ngnale looked forward to the visit she'd just scheduled. It always gave him pleasure to see her.

When Janice came in, Dr. Ngnale realized at once that things were different this time. She didn't look well: she was pale, had lost weight, and moved with a kind of weariness he'd never seen in her before.

What she told him deepened his concern. Yes, she said, she'd lost 12 pounds in just the past two months. Her appetite never came back after a bout of flu. Her husband noticed that she ate smaller and smaller portions. She was full after just a few bites, and, for all her husband's urging, she just couldn't eat any more. Her husband thought she might be having thyroid trouble or low blood sugar.

Toward the end of their conversation, Dr. Ngnale asked Janice if there had been any changes in her bowel or urinary functions. No, she told him, but she did have pains in her abdomen from time to time.

At this point, Dr. Ngnale had a focal point. Janice was suffering weight loss. Checking his records, the doctor found that she had lost not just the 12 pounds she mentioned but, since their last visit, 20 pounds in all. He also knew one important thing about the cause of that loss: Janice was suffering from what doctors call "early satiety." That's their way of describing the condition of people who feel full too fast—that is, before they've eaten enough to properly nourish themselves. Older people do surprisingly well under that condition,

SEER INCIDENCE AND U.S. DEATH RATES, † 1975–2002

Stomach Cancer, Both Sexes

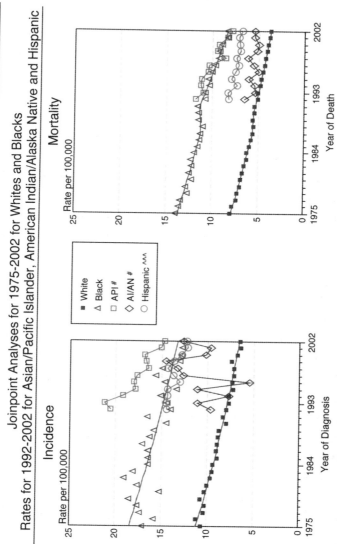

Joinpoint Analyses for 1975-2002 for Whites and Blacks
Rates for 1992-2002 for Asian/Pacific Islander, American Indian/Alaska Native and Hispanic

† Source: Incidence data for whites and blacks is from the SEER 9 areas (San Francisco, Connecticut, Detroit, Hawaii, Iowa, New Mexico, Seattle, Utah, Atlanta). Incidence data for Asian/Pacific Islanders, American Indian/Alaska Natives and Hispanics is from the SEER 13 Areas (SEER 9 Areas, San Jose-Monterey, Los Angeles, Alaska Native Registry and Rural Georgia). Mortality data is from NCHS public use data file for the total US. Rates are age-adjusted to the 2000 US Std Population (19 age groups - Census P25-1103).
Regression lines for whites and blacks are calculated using the Joinpoint Regression Program Version 3.0, April 2005, National Cancer Institute.
API = Asian/Pacific Islander. AI/AN = American Indian/Alaska Native.
^^^ Hispanic is not mutually exclusive from Whites, Blacks, Asian/Pacific Islanders, and American Indians/Alaska Natives. Incidence data for Hispanics excludes cases from Detroit, Hawaii, Alaska Native Registry and Rural Georgia. Mortality data for Hispanics excludes cases from Connecticut, Maine, Maryland, Minnesota, Oklahoma, New Hampshire, New York, North Dakota, and Vermont.

Surveillance, Epidemiology, and End Results (SEER) Program (www.seer.cancer.gov) SEER*Stat Database: Incidence - SEER 9 Regs Public-Use, Nov 2004 Sub (1973-2002), National Cancer Institute, DCCPS, Surveillance Research Program, Cancer Statistics Branch, released April 2005, based on the November 2004 submission.

and may experience it for a long time before they mention it to a doctor. Often, these older people, especially the tough, stoic ones, let the condition develop until pain finally brings them in.

Now early satiety, with its symptoms, is a common complaint, and abdominal pain is still more common. Such symptoms alone or in combination can point to a whole host of diseases. But most of them are benign and vanish soon.

Dr. Ngnale hoped that Janice simply needed some hormonal or other chemical rebalancing. He could provide that. Thyroid and diabetes would respond to medication. So, for that matter, would depression.

The only flaw in this line of thinking was that he would have noticed something during Janice's earlier visit if the trouble was thyroid or diabetes. As to depression, Janice denied feeling depressed, except for her concern about her condition. And she didn't act depressed, only appropriately worried.

That line of reasoning led Dr. Ngnale to a grim fact: weight loss, especially in an older person, may be a sign of cancer. Stomach cancer (also called gastric cancer) and pancreatic cancer were both high on the list of possibilities.

"Janice," he told her, "I can't know anything definite at this stage. We need to take tests. I'm going to arrange for you to get a CT scan of your abdomen. Also we're going to do some blood work. Finally—and I think we may be able to do this today—we'll take some x-ray pictures. With a little luck, I might be able to learn something about what's ailing you before the day's over."

AFRICAN AMERICANS AND STOMACH CANCER

Although stomach cancer is less common in the United States than in other parts of the world, each year almost 22,000 Americans are diagnosed with it. Here again, incidence and morality rates are higher for blacks than for whites, with incidence rates of

10.7/100,000 for whites and 17.7/100,000 for black men; and 5.0/100,000 for white women versus 9.0/100,000 for black women. Mortality rates are 12.8/100,000 for black men against 5.6/100,000 for white men.

INCIDENCE AND SURVIVAL

While stomach cancer is less common in the United States than in other parts of the world, the American Cancer Society estimates that 21,860 Americans (13,510 men and 8,350 women) will be diagnosed with it during 2005. An estimated 11,550 (6,770 men and 4,780 women) deaths from this type of cancer is projected for 2005. Two-thirds of people diagnosed with stomach cancer are older than 65. Five-year survival rates are about 23 percent, and if the cancer is discovered early, the figure rises to 60 percent.

ETIOLOGY

Doctors, like other scientists, like to use words that have specific, unmistakable meanings, and that fit into larger systems of classification. The word *etiology* refers to the causes of things. As doctors use it, it has to do with the causes of specific diseases.

But to get to causes we must get to *incidence*—that is, how widespread is the disease, and whether that spread is growing or declining. In the United States, fortunately, the incidence of gastric cancer has declined over the last several decades.

Causes of stomach cancer include:

- A diet high in salt
- A diet high in smoked foods, salted fish and meat, and pickled vegetables
- Age
- Sex—men are at highter risk than women.
- Consumption of meats cooked at high heat

- The bacteria called *Helicobacter pylori*, a risk factor that contributes to gastric cancer.

The problem with high-temperature cooking of meat is that it produces carcinogens (cancer-causing chemicals).

The most common type of gastric cancer is called adenocarcinoma, and, like peptic ulcer disease, it arises from the inside lining of the stomach. At first, the irritation is simply gastritis—that is, inflammation of the stomach. But it can progress into cancer. *Helicobacter pylori* is especially widespread in underdeveloped countries, where the incidence of gastric, or stomach, cancer is high.

In all these cancers of the GI tract, if the cancer progresses, it will eventually penetrate into and break through the wall of the gut. Once that happens, the lymph nodes become seeded with cancer cells. From that point on, the cancer can move easily to distant sites, commonly the liver or lung.

ANATOMY AND PHYSIOLOGY OF THE STOMACH

Anatomy means the way the parts are laid out—it comes from a Greek word meaning "to cut up." *Physiology* means how they work together and what comes out of that work. Let's look at the stomach from these perspectives.

As you know, our food must be converted into useable nutrients. That conversion takes place in the course of the journey the food takes from the mouth, where it enters, to the anus, where what the body hasn't used is excreted. In the course of that journey, fats, carbohydrates, and proteins are transported across the intestinal wall and absorbed into the bloodstream.

The process of digestion begins in the mouth, where mechanical chewing (mastication), along with the enzymes contained in saliva, breaks food into small pieces. Absorption itself takes place along the 22 feet of small bowel leading from the stomach to the large intestine. The stomach is a kind of midpoint between these processes. The stomach aids in the absorption process, but only in a limited way. Its basic function is as a storage site for food passing from the esophagus toward the small bowel.

The stomach itself is a thick-walled muscular pouch where food is ground into a small bolus, or small round mass. At the same time, the stomach is an environment especially vulnerable to disease.

One problem is that the high concentration of acids produced by the stomach can also damage the wall of the stomach itself. Damage to the interior lining of the stomach can expose the tissue itself to this highly concentrated acid. Over the course of time, this can result in peptic ulcer disease. Medications like aspirin or ibuprofen, as well as anti-inflammatory drugs, can sometimes cause such damage.

Besides peptic ulcers that can develop in the lining of the stomach and, sometimes, lead to cancer, there is a second problem. Where the esophagus joins the stomach, abrupt changes occur in the cell type lining this area. This junction (the *gastroesophageal,* or GE, junction) acts as a one-way valve to prevent the gastric contents from going back up into the lower esophagus. But if that valve operates imperfectly, heart burn or *reflux esophagitis* occurs. If that irritation becomes chronic—that is, goes on for a long time—it can lead to cancer, just as chronic inflammation of the stomach resulting from infection can.

DIAGNOSIS

Two days after her visit to Dr. Ngnale, Janice came to the hospital for a CT test. The test began when the radiologist had her drink a large cup of flavored x-ray dye. Janice drank the stuff without much trouble, though she'd have preferred a cup of coffee. As she drank, she noticed a glass panel at one end of the room where the radiologist was staring at her monitor while she talked to the young technician in the room with Janice.

Following the radiologist's instructions, the technician adjusted Janice's place on the CT scanner's hard table. As Janice lay there, the radiologist had her place her arms above her head and told her please to keep them there. This was to get them out of the way so they didn't interfere with the x-ray of her abdomen.

The technician had already placed an IV tube in Janice's arm, and now he began to infuse a contrast dye into her vein. Meanwhile, the table Janice lay on was moved into a large donut-shaped device—the CT scanner itself.

That's when Janice was almost overcome with a feeling of unpleasant warmth in her stomach that quickly turned to nausea. She thought she might vomit. But she got past that bad moment holding her breath several times, as the technician recommended.

While this was going on, the radiologist monitored the scanner. The target areas were Janice's abdomen and pelvis, and the radiologist paid especially close attention to the stomach and pancreas, where Dr. Ngnale in his notes had suggested the trouble might be. The CT scan takes small pictures of the target area. When some eighteen to twenty of these "slices" are taken and assembled, they give a pretty good picture of the entire area.

But because they are slices, they provide only sample pictures of the area. It is possible that a small tumor could fall between the slices. For that reason, when the radiologist came to the areas that Dr. Ngnale had warned her about, she adjusted the interval she was scanning to 3 mm. That meant more and smaller slices and greater detail.

As the monitor displayed each segment, the radiologist fine-tuned the picture. On the third slice, she saw what she was looking for—a defect protruding from the lumen (the inner space) of the stomach, clearly outlined by the dye. The defect, or lesion, appeared to involve the lower portion of the gastric wall, which appeared thickened. Later, the radiologist would study the pictures on a light box and write up her analysis. But for now, her work continued. She had found the primary problem, but she continued to study the rest of the abdomen.

She needed to find out if the cancer had spread to the liver or the surrounding lymph nodes. She also needed to know the size of the tumor itself, and whether it had gotten big enough to involve surrounding organs. Finally, she looked for evidence of free fluid within the abdomen, fluid that could contain (and spread) the cancer. When all that was done and she'd written up her notes, she paged Dr. Ngnale to describe her findings.

Her report read something like this. "A gastric cancer was confined to the end portion of the stomach with no evidence of spread to the liver or other structures. The lymph nodes surrounding the stomach were within the normal range, but they were slightly enlarged so they had to be considered suspicious."

Dr. Ngnale called Janice on the phone to tell her about the pathology report. "I'm sorry to tell you, Janice, that we found a tumor, and it's probably a cancer. Once we've taken a biopsy, we'll know for sure. There's some good news, too. As far as we can tell, the cancer hasn't spread to other organs."

Janice was numb. She handed the phone to her husband, Sam, and Sam asked the doctor to repeat what he'd told Janice. Dr. Ngnale did that, and added that they'd found the cause of her weight loss and fatigue. Sam took a deep breath and tried to compose himself.

"O.K., doctor. I've got a pretty good idea of where we are, then. But where do we go from here?"

"I need to talk first to the gastroenterologist I work with." The gastroenterologist, or stomach specialist, turned out to be our old acquaintance, Dr. Bambridge, who had operated successfully on Jack Tollen's colon cancer. "We'll set up an appointment," Dr. Ngnale continued. "Dr. Bambridge will need to do an endoscopy that lets him look inside the stomach. He'll also do the biopsy that will almost certainly confirm our diagnosis. It may also tell us a little more about the cancer. Once we have all that, we can make specific plans for treatment."

The next morning, Dr. Bambridge's nurse called to give instructions for preparations Janice would need to make for the endoscopy.

Sam took the message because Janice didn't trust herself to listen clearly. First the nurse told Sam how the test worked. The endoscope is a long, flexible tube that is inserted into the mouth, swallowed by the patient, and then gently manipulated into the stomach. It allows the physician to see the surfaces of the esophagus and stomach. It also is connected to a video monitor that displays an enlarged picture. And it takes photos along the way. Any areas that look suspicious get biopsied. Results of the biopsies come back in three or four days.

"O.K.," Sam said, "I'll tell Janice all that."

"Something else, Mr. Simmons," the nurse added. "We need Janice not to eat or drink anything after midnight of the day of the study. And you or somebody else will have to drive your wife to our office and back. We'll be giving Janice a sedative so she'll be comfortable, and she'll probably still be woozy when it's time to go home."

"Sure," Sam said. "I'll drive her myself. I can just take that day off."

"There's one more thing you and Mrs. Simmons should know," the nurse said. "This procedure won't be painful, but it can be a little uncomfortable. Sometimes it goes easier if the patient expects this in advance. It's also true that this procedure is invasive. Whenever we put foreign objects into people, complications can happen. In this case, the danger is that the instrument might perforate the esophagus or stomach. But I'm telling you this only so you'll know *all* the possibilities in advance. Complications are very rare, and to tell you the truth, in my ten years of working with Dr. Bambridge, I've never seen one. He's very good at what he does."

"Thanks, nurse. I guess that's all we can ask for—that and the help of God."

"I hear you, Mr. Simmons. One last thing. If Janice takes aspirin or any other blood thinners, she should stop using them. They can raise the risk of bleeding during the procedure."

Sam thanked the nurse, hung up the phone, and went to the living room where Janice was waiting. He reported what he'd learned, easing her mind as much as he could.

The next morning in Dr. Bambridge's office things went smoothly. Dr. Bambridge asked Janice a few questions. When she got tense, Sam helped her. Then Dr. Bambridge examined Janice's abdomen, and when that was done, he was ready to proceed with the endoscopy.

Preparations moved quickly. The assistant inserted a small catheter into one of Janice's veins, and attached her to several monitors. Then the inside of her mouth was sprayed with a numbing medication.

The next thing Janice realized was her husband standing next to the bed, talking in subdued tones with Dr. Bambridge. For a moment, Janice thought the exam hadn't begun, but then she felt soreness in her throat.

"Well, that wasn't as bad as I expected," she said, drowsily, to Sam. "No, you looked pretty comfortable," Sam said. After a minute or two, when Janice seemed more awake, Sam said, "Look at this." He handed her a picture of her stomach, pointing to what the doctors were pretty sure was the cancer. At first, the only thing Janice could make out was something that looked like a stream of blood. "Yes," Sam said, "that's just what it is—from where they took the biopsy sample. But look over here." Janice saw a small yellowish area that stood out from the smooth pink lining of the rest of the stomach. It looked small, but it looked like a sore. This was the cancer.

Dr. Bambridge could have studied the cancer in other ways. If he practiced where endoscopy wasn't available, he'd have done a barium contrast x-ray exam and gotten good results, though not as good as what the endoscopy provides. If he practiced where the very latest technique was available, he'd have done the endoscopy backed with ultrasound. The endoscopy itself would have worked as we described, but the ultrasound would allow a direct measurement of how deeply the cancer had penetrated into the wall.

Ultrasound is the only way to get that precise information, short of surgical resection.

While Janice waited to hear from Dr. Bambridge's office about what treatment she'd need, she went through a kind of initiation experience. Until she'd been diagnosed with it, she'd known nothing about gastric cancer. The only cancer in her immediate circle was her sister-in-law's breast cancer, from which she seemed to be recovering nicely.

Janice found something about other kinds of cancer in almost every magazine she picked up. But about her illness, Janice found almost nothing. There seemed to be no races for a cure for stomach cancer.

WAITING FOR THE PATHOLOGY REPORT

While they waited to hear the results of the lab tests, including blood samples, Janice and Sam spent an anxious time. Two weeks had slipped by since Dr. Ngnale had first given her the bad news. While she waited for a call from the doctor's office, she and Sam mulled over the many questions they had in their minds:

- Is it cancer for sure? The doctors all said, didn't they, that they can't be certain till they get the biopsy results.
- If it is cancer, will I need surgery?
- Can they get it all with surgery?
- Is my life in danger?
- What should we say to the children, and when?

And Sam had a special set of questions of his own, so frightening he could hardly think about them. They all came back to the one big and terrible question: *What would I do if Janice died? No, it won't happen, I'm sure it won't happen. But what would I do?* There couldn't be any answer to that one. It just kept haunting him like a buzzing fly that wouldn't go away.

Then the call came that they'd been waiting for and dreading. It was Dr. Bambridge telling them that he'd made an appointment for

Janice with a surgeon. She'd need to talk to the surgeon, hear what he had to say. She and Sam would have to decide whether to go along with the treatment the surgeon recommended. Janice said that she felt she was being pushed step by step into a den where a wild animal waited.

"No, it's not like that," Sam said. "We're going to tame this beast." Janice took real comfort from his confident eyes.

TALKING TO THE SURGEON

Janice brought her x-rays to Dr. Barnes's office. The surgeon asked her again questions she'd answered before, about her weight loss, about previous surgery (she'd had none). After he was done with his exam, he asked her what she knew about her condition.

Janice knew a great deal, but she found it hard to talk about it to strangers. Even to herself it was difficult to say that she almost certainly had cancer in the stomach. But she did say it, and then Dr. Barnes told her and Sam a little more about the treatment the doctor recommended.

Janice and Sam were shaken to find that the doctor wasn't talking about a cure. "We want to remove the cancer we can see, of course," he said. "That means surgery. But we can't be sure we'll get it all. Your cancer has penetrated the wall of the stomach and may involve the lymph nodes. This means that we want to follow up the surgery with chemotherapy to control that possible secondary growth. Depending on how things look at that stage, we may want to use radiation as well."

"Just what are you saying?" Sam asked. "If you can't cure Janice, what *can* you do?"

"By performing the surgery, and following it up with chemotherapy and possibly radiation, we can delay the recurrence of the cancer. No, we probably can't cure it. So we'll be treating it as a chronic condition, keeping a sharp eye on it, and fighting it battle by battle. Janice can have periods of reasonably good health. And there's always a chance, if we can keep the cancer at bay for five years or more, that it *won't* return."

Now that Janice and Sam knew that there would probably be no miraculous cure, they were ready for the fight. For the moment, that meant asking questions like these:

- How far has the cancer spread?
- Were they likely to find, once they were inside, that the cancer had spread to places not shown on the tests?
- How long would the operation take?
- How long before Janice's stomach and intestine healed well enough to start working again?
- How would they feed Janice till then, and what could she eat after she'd recovered? (Dr. Barnes told her that she'd be on an IV for a few days, then on a liquid diet, then, gradually, on a solid diet.)

Sam had heard that surgeons can spread the cancer by letting air in during the operation, and he wanted to know if this were true.

"No," Dr. Barnes assured him. "This rumor started when our detection tests were still fairly primitive, and the only way to find anything out was to go inside. Because we didn't have a good way to spot the disease early, surgeons most often operated on patients with advanced disease. Since the cancer was inoperable, they could only do a biopsy, just to confirm the diagnosis. Postoperative patients in late-stage cancers often *did* die soon after the operation, and that's why people sometimes thought that the operation had caused the spread of cancer—by letting the air in. It's simply not true."

Dr. Barnes also told Janice and Sam how the actual operation would go. Once he'd made the incision and exposed the stomach, he would explore the abdominal cavity. Then he'd remove the primary tumor—the one spotted already—and send that to the pathologist.

He'd pay special attention to the margins of resection—that is, to the edges of the parts of the stomach he sewed back together. He had to be confident that he hadn't left cancer cells behind. So he would examine these two margins microscopically.

COMPLICATIONS FROM SURGERY

At this point, Janice wanted to know how much risk there was of her dying directly or indirectly as a result of the operation itself. Here Dr. Barnes was reassuring. The great majority of his patients make a good recovery, and within six to eight weeks. In a small percent of all cases, complications like internal bleeding or infection can develop, and they make the recovery period longer. Some people have internal bleeding, sometimes there's an infection, and some people take longer than others before their intestines work, or they develop blockages in their intestines.

In a few cases, people experience diarrhea and cramps, and occasional bouts of vomiting. What happens to them is that food enters the intestines too fast and is dumped into the bowel. This tends to overload the small intestine. Those people have to go on pretty strict diets. But, again, such cases are rare.

Older patients who have previous medical problems unrelated to the cancer are most at risk from complications. So are patients with advanced disease.

But Janice felt better when he reassured her that, even though she'd lost weight, because her health was excellent except for the cancer, he was as confident as a surgeon can be in an uncertain world that she'd come through this with flying colors and that she and Sam would still have plenty of good life to live together.

SURGERY

What Janice remembered most clearly about the day of the surgery was the time just before it. She felt rushed, hurried from one place to another. There was more paper work to fill out, and a nurse asked her questions she'd already answered in other offices several times before. But Dr. Barnes had told her to expect all this. "It's the nurse's job to make sure you're ready for surgery, so there won't be any last-minute slipups," he said. There was also some last-minute lab work done on her, and the anesthesiologist came by to ensure that her vital signs were all strong.

The next thing Janice felt was the wave of anxiety that came over her as she entered the operating room. The fact that the air felt icy cold didn't help quiet her nerves. Neither did the sight of all these masked people busy over equipment and laying out instruments. She was glad when Dr. Barnes, whom she hadn't recognized under his mask, put a hand on her shoulder and said a few reassuring words.

Now they were putting what Janice later called "a lot of fastenings" on her: an intravenous catheter that would stay in until she was able to eat normally again; a blood pressure cuff on her arm; pads on her chest for heart monitoring.

That was all Janice remembered because now the anesthesiologist gently placed a mask over her mouth. As she took long, deep breaths, she heard some gentle words of comfort. Those were the last words she'd hear until she awakened.

Now last-minute preparations moved quickly. A tube was placed in her trachea so that during the operation her breathing could be controlled by a ventilator. Then a catheter was placed in the bladder to measure the urine output during the surgery. A temperature probe was inserted, and another tube was positioned in the stomach through the nose.

Now she was ready for Dr. Barnes. He made an incision straight down the middle of the abdomen. Once inside, he explored the abdominal cavity. No, no signs of cancer except for the tumor they'd discovered originally. Dr. Barnes resected a major portion of the stomach, which included the tumor. The remainder of the stomach he connected to the small bowel. Then he closed the incision. It had been a routine procedure, and he was finished in a little over two hours.

AFTER THE OPERATION

While Dr. Barnes was telling Sam and the children that everything had gone well, Janice was in the recovery room being closely monitored. That monitoring would continue for the next three to four days. If complications were to develop, that's when it would happen. In the meantime, everything was done to keep Janice as comfortable as possible.

Sam wanted to know more about whether chemotherapy and radiation would be needed, but Dr. Barnes wanted to redirect his concern to the present. There would be plenty of time to discuss and formulate future treatment plans. For now, recovery from surgery was the priority. "I find it best, for myself, to take things one day at a time," he told Sam, "and that's the medicine I'd prescribe for you too, Sam." Sam said that he'd try.

"In a few days," the surgeon added, "we'll know more about the extent of the disease. Remember, cure is difficult. Our aim is to keep the disease under control. I'll be talking with you in the next few days about the choices we have here."

Janice made an excellent recovery. Six days after the operation, she was walking, though a bit hesitantly and painfully. She was also able to eat small meals. She'd be coming home in a day or two, though it would be another four weeks before she started to regain her strength.

In the meantime, the much awaited pathology report came in. The description of the resected specimen ran some three pages. As expected, it was an adenocarcinoma of the stomach that had extended into the wall of the stomach and penetrated through the wall to involve the outside of the wall. Three lymph nodes were involved with cancer. The margins of the resection were clear of cancer.

That was the picture in a nutshell. Dr. Barnes knew now that the cancer was advanced. Statistically, Janice's chance for cure was poor, even with the help of chemotherapy and radiation. The goal had to be delaying any recurrence. As things stood, the disease was micro-scopic. To keep it in check and to keep it from coming back—that was the route to promise Janice the best quality of life and the best chance of survival.

His interview with Sam and Janice wasn't easy. Though he'd told them what to prepare for, emotionally that was difficult for them. After all, didn't Janice feel a lot better? Didn't the doctor say that there were no visible signs of metastasis?

"Yes," Dr. Barnes said, "that's true. But the lymph node involve-ment means that, even though we can't see it, there are microscopic deposits, which represent what we call occult (hidden) metastasis.

"What it boils down to, I'm afraid, is that you have to see still another doctor. I've made an appointment for you with Dr. Perez. He's what we call a medical oncologist—a doctor who specializes in the treatment of cancer. He'll help you choose between chemother-apy or radiation or a combination, and he'll carry out the treatment plan you decide on.

"The oncologist will also tell you about clinical trials where researchers are studying the relative advantages and disadvantages of the treatments now in use. He may recommend that you get into one of those trials. That will be up to you, of course, but if you go that way you'll be assured that you will get one of the best available kinds of treatments. And you'll also know that through your treatment, researchers are learning things that may help other people. Naturally, we won't start any new treatment until you're fully recovered from the surgery."

Surgery alone can cure only early cancers.

For Janice and Sam, this was a bad moment. Both of them felt overwhelmed by negative emotions—first, fear, then disbelief and anger. But with Dr. Barnes's help, they calmed down. They knew that they had a fight on their hands and that it might go on for a long time. They knew that they'd have to learn to live with fears, yet still keep hope alive. But they'd been in tough spots before, and they knew that, with each other's help, they could do what this difficult stage of their lives demanded of them.

CHEMOTHERAPY

As you know, surgery alone can cure only early cancers. When, as in Janice's case, there's lymph node involvement and a high probability of spread, or where the primary cancer is large or has invaded surrounding tissues, chemotherapy is usually used.

Janice's cancer had penetrated the wall of the stomach, and three of her lymph nodes contained cancer cells. This meant, to the doctors, that hers was a stage III cancer. Nobody likes to think of himself or herself as part of a statistical sample, but statistics can help us understand certain things. For instance, it told Dr. Barnes and Dr. Perez that only 15 percent of patients at Janice's stage were cured. As to the remaining 85 percent, they had cancer in them that present medical procedures couldn't detect. Yet it had to be treated.

How do we treat something we can't see but must assume exists? The answer lies in the circulatory system (blood flow) that provides nourishment to all cells of the body. In chemotherapy, drugs are injected into the vein. This allows the chemical agents to be carried through the entire circulatory system to all areas of the body, interfering with the process of cellular multiplication by which cancer spreads.

Chemotherapy is used when there is lymph node involvement and a high probability of cancer spread.

Chemotherapy is a systemic therapy, as opposed to surgery and radiotherapy, which are local therapies. These latter concentrated on the diseased area; the former, we might say, attacks the transportation system used by the disease.

Unfortunately, gastric cancer is especially resistant to chemical agents. That's why cancer often recurs in the remaining stomach. Because that area is well defined, medical oncologists often recommend radiation therapy in addition to the chemo. Early findings suggest that it helps decrease the recurrence rate.

Many other kinds of drugs used in chemo work in different ways. Usually, several of these drugs are used together. That raises the odds that one of them will be effective. Chemotherapy requires strong drugs, and they have strong side effects; common among these are:

- Nausea
- Lethargy
- Diarrhea
- Infection
- Anemia.

Because every cell of the body is exposed to chemotherapy, damage to normal cells occurs. Cells that normally divide—hair cells, blood elements, cells that line the intestinal tract—are particularly affected. Because these drugs are toxic, maximum doses must be limited. Medical oncologists walk a fine line between giving too much chemotherapy or not enough.

Chemotherapy can last up to several months. Because the therapies use multiple drugs, the time frames can get complicated. But the general rule is that intravenous treatment is given every three to four weeks. If the chemotherapy is aimed at occult metastasis, it will go on for as long as six months. Clinical studies help determine when to stop treatment.

If metastatic disease has actually developed—say, in the liver or lung—the aim of chemotherapy will be to prevent the growth or to decrease the size of the mass. In such cases, x-ray will commonly be used to follow up chemotherapy. If the tumor continues to grow or new masses appear while treatment is going on, the treatment obviously is not working, and a change in plan is needed.

Cancer patients need to be followed for life. The risk of recurrent disease is always present, though after five to ten years it declines. Follow-up exams include endoscopy, blood work, and CT scans.

As to Janice, three years after surgery, chemotherapy, and radiation therapy, she's doing well. Her doctors haven't found reason to start new treatments. Janice and Sam have adjusted to the lifestyle that Dr. Barnes recommended to Sam after the operation: one day at a time. Very often they have fine days.

IN A NUTSHELL

Incidence:
About 22,000 new cases are diagnosed each year

Causes:
- A diet high in salt
- A diet high in smoked or pickled meats
- Consumption of meats cooked at high heat
- The bacteria called *Heliobacter pylori*, a risk factor that contributes to gastric cancer.

Prevention:
Avoid diets high in salt. Avoid eating meat cooked over high heat.

Diagnosis:
Be alert to:
- Early satiety
- Weight loss
- Abdominal pain
- Fatigue.

Your doctor will perform:
- CT scan
- Endoscopy
- Biopsy.

Treatment:
Surgery, followed by radiation and/or chemical therapy.

Prognosis:
Good if caught early, poor in later stages.

SEVENTEEN

Pancreatic Cancer

THE CASE OF DR. CHARLES BYSON

CHARLEY HAD BEEN MY DENTIST for years, and a good one. He was a hearty, good-natured man who always seemed to bubble over with good health and good spirit. When he called me, I could tell at once from the tone of his voice that this wasn't a social occasion. He was obviously troubled.

In the past few days, he'd noticed some disturbing changes in his health. It began on a Wednesday while he was brushing his teeth: that's when he saw that the whites of his eyes were yellow. In the next day or two, he saw other changes. His urine had a peculiar brown tint, and his feces were clay colored. Charley had a vague recollection from the pathology course he took in dental school that all these symptoms were related to the pancreas. What he couldn't remember was whether these were symptoms of inflammation of the pancreas (*pancreatitis*), or diabetes, or of cancer.

These symptoms told me that Charley was in trouble. Yellow eyes, green urine, and clay-colored stools are the diagnostic triad of obstructive cancer. If the patient felt pain as well, these symptoms might point to a less serious disease of the pancreas. But Charley didn't mention pain.

When Charley came to my office, he was jovial and looked healthy enough. He'd lost 10 pounds in the past month, though, and he felt a bit weakened, he said. Of course, I could see at once that his eyes were yellow.

When I examined him physically, I felt a mass in the upper right side of his abdomen. It wasn't tender. I thought it was probably a distended gallbladder caused by blocked bile ducts.

Tests showed us a little more, and what they showed confirmed my fears. There was a tumor in the pancreas. Although there were no other masses, in this case, that fact didn't give me much relief. I knew that pancreatic cancer was very aggressive. I also knew that the survival rate was poor.

Charley and I agreed that he needed surgery. I made it clear that the best I could hope for was to extend his life. With or without surgery, the vast majority of patients diagnosed with the disease die within two years of the diagnosis, even when they have surgery.

In Charley's case, the surgery was extensive. The operation, called a *Whipple* after the surgeon who first performed it, involved the removal of that part of the pancreas that contained the tumor, as well as parts of the stomach and intestine, gallbladder and bile ducts. We discovered that three lymph nodes were involved in the cancer.

Charley lived for almost two years before he died of generalized metastasis. For eighteen months of that time, he was without pain, able to work and to resume his other normal activities. The last time I saw him when he was close to death, he thanked me for those days. "They were the richest in my life, Doc, each day a jewel."

ANATOMY AND FUNCTION OF THE PANCREAS

The 6-inch long pancreas lies across the back of the abdomen behind the stomach. One end of the pancreas, the head, is wide, the other, the tail, narrow. The midsection is called the body.

FIGURE 25

ANATOMY OF THE PANCREAS

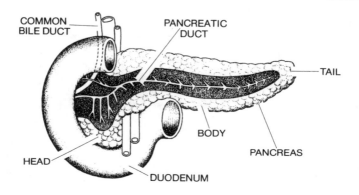

The pancreas has two main functions. First, it produces several hormones, including insulin, which, secreted into the bloodstream, controls the body's use of sugar. Second, the pancreas secretes juices that contain proteins, called enzymes, that help digest food. The main pancreatic duct joins the bile duct from the liver and gallbladder.

PANCREATIC CANCER

Being black is one of the risk factors for pancreatic cancer listed by the National Cancer Society. Pancreatic cancer is one of the leading causes of death in the United States and the world, with an estimated 33,000 deaths in the U.S. alone. Again, the five-year survival rate is better for whites than for blacks. For white males it is 5.3 percent; for black males, 3.4 percent. The picture is worse for women: white women, 4.6 percent black women 5.5 percent. Pancreatic cancer is almost never caught early. In over 90 percent of patients at the time of diagnosis, it has already spread beyond the pancreas. Ninety-five percent of these patients die of the disease. Few survive two years, with or without surgery.

In thirty-four years of practice, I have performed eighteen Whipples, and not one of these survived five years. In fewer than 10

FIGURE 26

SEER INCIDENCE AND U.S. DEATH RATES,[†] 1975–2002

Pancreas Cancer, Both Sexes

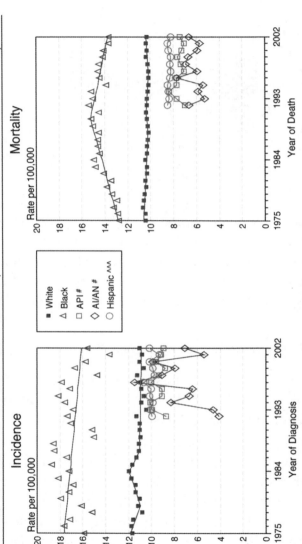

Joinpoint Analyses for 1975-2002 for Whites and Blacks
Rates for 1992-2002 for Asian/Pacific Islander, American Indian/Alaska Native and Hispanic

† Source: Incidence data for whites and blacks is from the SEER 9 areas (San Francisco, Connecticut, Detroit, Hawaii, Iowa, New Mexico, Seattle, Utah, Atlanta).
Incidence data for Asian/Pacific Islanders, American Indian/Alaska Natives and Hispanics is from the SEER 13 Areas (SEER 9 Areas, San Jose-Monterey, Los Angeles,
Alaska Native Registry and Rural Georgia). Mortality data is from NCHS public use data file for the total US.
Rates are age-adjusted to the 2000 US Std Population (19 age groups - Census P25-1103).
Regression lines for whites and blacks are calculated using the Joinpoint Regression Program Version 3.0, April 2005, National Cancer Institute.
API = Asian/Pacific Islander. AI/AN = American Indian/Alaska Native.
^^^ Hispanic is not mutually exclusive from Whites, Blacks, Asian/Pacific Islanders, and American Indians/Alaska Natives. Incidence data for Hispanics excludes
cases from Detroit, Hawaii, Alaska Native Registry and Rural Georgia. Mortality data for Hispanics excludes cases from Connecticut, Maine, Maryland, Minnesota,
Oklahoma, New Hampshire, New York, North Dakota, and Vermont.

Surveillance, Epidemiology, and End Results (SEER) Program (www.seer.cancer.gov) SEER*Stat Database: Incidence - SEER 9 Regs Public-Use,
Nov 2004 Sub (1973-2002), National Cancer Institute, DCCPS, Surveillance Research Program, Cancer Statistics Branch, released April 2005,

percent of these cases did I even resect in the hope of cure. Too often, by the time I saw it, the cancer had spread too far, beyond any chance of cure.

CAUSES

You won't be surprised to learn that cigarette smokers are at two to three times the risk as nonsmokers. Diabetics, too, are at special risk, developing pancreatic cancer twice as often as nondiabetics. Some studies suggest that steady exposure to petroleum may also be a risk factor. Other studies suggest that a high-fat diet adds to the risks.

Cigarette smokers are at two to three times the risk as nonsmokers.

PREVENTION

Among the courses of action you can take to help prevent pancreatic cancer are the following:

- Don't smoke.
- Eat a low-fat diet.
- Eat a diet rich in fruits and vegetables.

SYMPTOMS

Pancreatic cancer is called a "silent" disease because symptoms don't usually occur until the cancer has already spread beyond the pancreas. What we hope for is that the cancer will grow inward and block the bile duct, thus causing jaundice early. Whether this happens early or, as in Charley's case, late, the symptoms are the ones you're already familiar with:

- Yellow eyes
- Green urine

- Clay-colored stools.

These symptoms develop because the bile produced in the liver cannot enter the intestines but is blocked by the tumor. When that happens, the bile backs up and spills into the bloodstream. This means that less bile gets into the stools, causing them to be clay colored. Further, the spillover of bile into the bloodstream causes the bile to stain all tissues green, hence the yellow-green whites of the eyes. Bile also passes in the urine, causing it to be dark green.

DIAGNOSIS

In most cases, the patient will be the first to suspect something is wrong. Should the three symptoms, or sudden weight loss, occur, see your doctor at once. Once pains develops, it is almost always too late for effective treatment.

After listening to your medical history, your doctor will give you a physical exam. Following this, you will be given several tests, probably by a gastroenterologist, or specialist in diseases of the stomach and intestine:

- A blood test called a *bilirubin*, which measures the bile in the blood and urine
- A CT scan, which can detect the spread of cancer to vital structures
- An ultrasound, which can determine the presence or absence of gallstones, a far less serious condition
- A test called the ERPC (a special kind of endoscopy), which allows the doctor to pass a small tube into the bile duct, inject dye, and take a picture
- X-rays, which can provide images of both the pancreatic and bile ducts
- Another kind of dye-assisted x-ray called a *transhepatic cholangiogram*, which determines whether the bile duct is blocked
- An *angiogram*, an x-ray of the blood vessels, which helps

decide whether to attempt surgery; if the tumor has invaded blood vessels, surgery is virtually impossible

- Laparoscopy, by means of a fiber-optic tube inserted surgically into the abdomen, which shows whether there are metastases of the lining of the abdomen or surface of the liver.

Final diagnosis, as always will depend on biopsy of the tumor. But because the visualizing techniques have become so sophisticated, some surgeons, if symptoms also indicate pancreatic cancer, will proceed with surgery without a biopsy.

TREATMENT

The only curative therapy for pancreatic cancer is surgery, and that works only if the tumor is discovered early. Most patients opt for surgery even when the cancer is in later stages. Surgery offers longer life for patients with pancreatic cancer. It also offers the only hope.

The surgery is very extensive, but it often assures the patient a year or two during which symptoms are relieved and the patient can get back to a normal life. There is always the chance of cure, but, even without it, my own patients have always expressed gratitude for the extended life surgery gave them.

You'll wish to bring questions when you talk with your gastroenterologist about treatment. Write them down and bring the paper with you. Here are some examples:

- How certain is the diagnosis?
- At what stage is the cancer?
- What are the benefits and risks of surgery?
- What other treatment options are open?
- Are there clinical trials I might enter?
- What are my chances of being cured—or of having a year or two of reasonably normal life?

THE COMPLICATIONS OF SURGERY

The surgical operation is extensive: it removes the diseased portion of the pancreas, part of the stomach and intestine, the gallbladder, and a portion of the common duct. Your organs are then joined back together: stomach to intestine, bile duct to intestine, pancreas to intestine.

The most immediate complications that can result from the surgery are internal bleeding and leakage of the hookup between pancreas and intestine. Such leakage can cause serious infection. Reoperations may be required to correct that complication.

The mortality rate of the surgery alone is in the range of 5 percent.

When surgery is inadvisable because the cancer is widespread, a nonsurgical procedure that allows a bypass of the obstructed bile duct may offer some relief.

IN A NUTSHELL

Incidence:
According to the National Cancer Society, approximately 33,700 Americans will be diagnosed with pancreatic cancer, and 32,300 will die of it. It is the fourth leading cause of cancer death.

Cause:
Unknown

Risk Factors:
- Cigarette smoking
- Diabetes
- High-fat diet
- Long-term exposure to petroleum.

Prevention:
Don't smoke; eat a low-fat, high-fiber diet rich in fruits and vegetables.

Diagnosis:
Be alert to:
- Jaundice
- Chronic itching
- Weight loss
- Abdominal or mid back pain in late stages.

Your doctor will use:
- CT scan
- ERCP
- Ultrasound
- Biopsy.

EIGHTEEN

Head and Neck Cancers

SHAWN'S STORY

SHAWN WASN'T A MAN to go to the dentist unless he needed to. But one day in June he complained to his wife about a lump he felt with his tongue on the floor of his mouth, behind his front teeth. Alice looked. Yes, she could see it, and didn't like what she saw: a small red, open sore. This time she drove Shawn to the dentist herself. What the dentist said, after a brief examination, was: "I don't like what I see, Shawn. It's probably nothing worse than a swollen salivary gland that's become inflamed. But we need to get you over to an ENT surgeon. That's ear, nose, and throat. He'll want to do tests. I don't believe in taking chances with these things."

That's how Shawn learned that he had cancer of the mouth. The good news was that it turned out to be stage I. Shawn was one of the happy few who get lucky.

THE ORAL CAVITY

Before we get into the characteristics, diagnosis, and treatment of cancers of the head and neck, we need to tell you something about the area in which they occur.

The oral cavity and pharynx are lined with a smooth, moist surface. Saliva is continuously produced there by salivary glands. The lower jaw, or mandible, supports the teeth and is where various muscles, including the tongue, are attached.

The palate is the bony roof of the oral cavity. In the front of the oral cavity is the hard palate. Where it extends into the pharynx, it becomes the soft palate.

A large part of the oral cavity is surrounded by bone. That bone protects the delicate structures of the face, but it also gives shape to the face.

SELF-EXAMINING FOR CANCERS OF THE HEAD AND NECK

Cancers of the head and neck have a common property: they grow in a kind of scaly tissue called *squamous tissue*, which is the outermost layer of skin. They may occur in the oral cavity, as in Shawn's case, or in the parts of the upper digestive tract called the *pharynx* and hypopharynx, or in the part of the upper respiratory tract called the *larynx*.

Such cancers of the head and neck are among the more preventable ones. Although these cancers are often found late, and sometimes too late, they ought to be found early. You can do this simple self-examination. Here's how it works:

- Stand in front of a well-lit mirror.
- Examine carefully your lips, as much of your tongue as you can see, the inside lining of your cheek, the roof of your mouth as far back as you can see, and the gums.
- If you wear dentures, take them out before you begin your self-

examination. Cancer inside the mouth often arises from the alveolar ridge, that ridge of hard tissue the lower denture rests on.

You will be looking for persistent open sores, and also lumps, under the tongue, on the gums, or on the roof of the mouth. If you find such sores or lumps, see your doctor at once.

MEDICAL EXAMINATION OF OTHER AREAS

Your doctor will examine first the areas we just described. The rest of his or her exam will require procedures you won't be able to perform for yourself.

- Using a tongue depressor, the doctor will get a look at your pharynx (at the back of the throat), and at the same time examine the tonsils, the back part of your tongue, and soft palate.
- Using a small, angled mirror, the doctor will then examine your pharynx and your larynx (voice box). Because the back of the throat is sensitive to foreign objects, he'll desensitize it with a spray that numbs it. That prevents gagging or vomiting.
- After he's completed the visual examination, the doctor will feel for sores or lumps or bumps that may be hidden under the surface of the oral cavity. (Shawn's tumor started beneath the surface, and had he been examined, his dentist or physician would have discovered it at that stage.)
- The doctor will also feel for sores or lumps in the salivary glands, which are located under the tongue, as well as the gums and the roof of the mouth.
- Next, he'll examine your neck, feeling the thyroid gland, the lymph nodes in the neck, and salivary glands. He'll note any enlargement, possible tumor, or tenderness. (Enlarged lymph nodes can have causes other than cancer. These include tuberculosis, HIV/AIDS, syphilis, as well as mononucleosis.)
- At some point in the physical examination, the physician will listen with a stethoscope to the rush of blood through the carotid

artery, the one in the neck. Abnormalities there produce a "swooshing" sound that may indicate heart or vascular disease.

One final note about what your doctor will look for. Certain cancers not directly related to the head and neck—like lymphoma, lung cancer, gastrointestinal (GI) tract cancer—can spread to the cervical nodes in your neck. Indeed, those nodes are a major site for capturing cancer cells or bacteria that have escaped into the lymphatic system. So your doctor will examine this area if he or she is checking you after treatment for one of these cancers. That is one way to monitor whether the cancer has spread into the lymphatic system, where it can be carried to other organs.

SIGNS AND SYMPTOMS OF CANCERS OF THE HEAD AND NECK

Recall that Shawn first noted a small, red, open sore under his tongue. He hadn't noticed it earlier because it didn't hurt and interfere with chewing or eating. This points to a principal problem in the diagnosis of cancers in the oral cavity: because they rarely interfere with normal body functions, they are usually ignored. Only when they cause an interruption in body function or, as in Shawn's case, when one is lucky enough to detect them early with the eye or tongue, are they likely to be noticed. Once they've been noticed, it's important that you seek medical attention. Although such sores can simply be canker sores, it's best to let your doctor determine whether they are that or something more serious.

If Shawn had not caught the sore when he did, it might have become tender or painful. It might also have swelled or bled. By that time, the cancer would have been in a late stage. If the cancer were allowed to grow still further, problems with chewing and swallowing, and even changes in the voice, could become symptoms.

Speaking generally, the first sign of cancer in the oral cavity is a change in the color of its lining (the mucosa), a sore, a lump, or bleeding from the lips, mouth, or gums. Because the change in color is subtle, and can show itself in either red or white patches, the examining physician needs especially good lighting—and a high degree of suspicion as well.

If such patches are left untreated, they can become nonhealing ulcers, or, in some cases, the ulcers will scab and heal, but then return soon after. This shouldn't be confused with ulcerations caused by poorly fitting dentures. That condition is easily treatable. Nevertheless, in such cases, the physician must be the one to rule out cancer.

Ulcerations deep in the throat can lead to blood-tinged sputum or pain. Any ulcer that doesn't heal within two weeks needs to be biopsied.

Such an ulceration can also develop on the tongue or floor of the mouth. Here it begins as a small mass that may be attributed to having accidentally bitten one's tongue. But in the case of potentially cancerous ulcerations, the mass will expand and tear, causing pain.

Tongue cancer usually starts at the side of the tongue, rarely on the top. Cancers that arise on the floor of the mouth are located under the tongue, just in back of the lower gum. When cancers do occur in the back of the tongue, they interfere with the tongue's mobility, making speech difficult.

A special problem posed by cancers in the head and neck is that this area has an abundant blood supply as well as an extensive lymphatic system. Injuries to this area can cause extensive bleeding. Sometimes infections or cancer itself can injure tissue here and cause bleeding.

The lymphatic system, the immune system's main line of defense, can also be a gathering place for cancer cells. When invasive cells, the result of cancer or infection, accumulate here, the lymph glands in the neck will enlarge. Infection in this area is called *lymphadenopathy* (meaning enlarged lymph nodes), and its most common cause is a cold or flu, with accompanying symptoms of sore throat, temperature, fever, earaches, and muscle aches.

Such symptoms will usually fade under treatment with antibiotics. But if they last for as long as two weeks, further examination becomes necessary. Symptoms like these can also be caused by cancer of the pharynx.

Remember that Shawn's dentist at first thought that the lump on the floor of his mouth might be a swollen salivary gland—glands located under the tongue but also scattered throughout the oral cavity. Infections can develop in these glands, causing pain and swelling.

Though Shawn's dentist believed that such a condition might be Shawn's problem, he also knew that Shawn had been a heavy smoker for a long time. That's why he knew that cancer was a strong possibility and referred him to an ear, nose, and throat (ENT) surgeon (also known as an *otolaryngologist*).

SHAWN GETS EXAMINED

Shawn's experience in the surgeon's examination room was a kind of summary of what you've already learned. After listening to a history of Shawn's complaints, Dr. Griswold, the ENT man, began his physical examination. Here his tools were his eyes and his hands.

The doctor began simply by looking at the oral cavity, and feeling the mass in the floor of Shawn's mouth. Then he felt for swollen lymph nodes in Shawn's neck. Although he didn't find any, he knew that this didn't necessarily mean that the cancer hadn't begun to penetrate there.

At this point, Dr. Griswold needed to use instruments. He numbed Shawn's nose and throat to prevent the gag reflex. Then he inserted a flexible laryngoscope, the basic diagnostic instrument used in such cases.

Sometimes a rigid instrument must be used in order to obtain a wider view and a clearer image of the structures within the pharynx. That involves a more difficult procedure because the instrument, besides being rigid, is larger. But the rigid instrument also allows the physician to obtain biopsy samples or to remove small tumors.

In Shawn's case, because the only visible abnormality was the small mass in his mouth, the rigid laryngoscope wasn't needed. Instead, Dr. Griswold took a biopsy sample of the mass. Lab results confirmed that it was cancerous.

The doctor's next job was to document the size of the tumor. For larger cancers that involved deeper structures of the neck, he would have used x-ray, perhaps supported by a computer scan that would show if the tumor was close to major blood vessels, nerves, and bones. Such tests are the basis of surgical strategy.

STAGING CANCERS OF THE HEAD AND NECK

The symptom for staging head and neck cancers is simple: they are classified as early, intermediate, or advanced. As with other cancers, the stage is determined according to the size of the tumor, the involvement or noninvolvement of the lymph nodes, and whether the cancer has spread (metastasized) to other areas of the body. Again, as with other cancers, the earlier the stage of the cancer, the better the prognosis. Once a doctor has established the stage of the disease, he or she can also begin to talk about treatment options and about whether the patient has a reasonable chance for a long life to come.

At the same time, prediction of outcomes is not something that can be done by formulas. Exceptional recoveries may be exceptional, but they occur. We will talk in more detail later in this book about living with cancer. But I've found, through my own experience and the experiences of others, that the best approach is to go through treatment. I don't pretend that that is an easy balance to maintain, but it is certainly the best medicine the patient can bring to the treatment process.

TREATMENT OF HEAD AND
NECK CANCERS

The mainstays of treatment for head and neck cancers are surgery and radiation. For early stage cancers, both treatments get good results—over 90 percent of stage I cancers have survival rates greater than five years. Here, the choice of treatment will depend in part on the strengths of the available treatment center. Some hospitals and treatment centers don't have radiation facilities at all. Others don't have sufficient staff experienced in surgical therapy or rehabilitation.

For small cancers of the lip, the anterior (front) of the tongue, palate, or cheek, surgical resection is often used. It has several advantages: the treatment can be completed in one setting, and the functional and cosmetic results are excellent—that is, your mouth will work as well as it always did, and your beauty will shine just as brightly.

When it comes to the larger cancers, treatment becomes more complicated and choices more difficult. Large cancers of the oral activity or pharynx may require partial tongue or lower jawbone (mandible) resection. Such treatment may result not only in significant speech and swallowing impairment, but also in disfigurement. It may also require a permanent breathing tube and, if swallowing becomes seriously impaired, a feeding tube. Some patients suffer partial or total loss of voice.

In cases of small oral cancer—and this generally applies when the cancer is smaller than 4 cm—the physician may decide that radiation therapy alone can achieve the same results as surgery and will recommend it. But radiation poses problems of its own. For one thing, it requires considerable commitment from the patient: the treatment goes on for six weeks, five days each week. During that period, the patient's life will be pretty much on hold.

There are other problems as well. Radiation therapy destroys cancer, but it destroys normal tissue, too. The better the radiation therapist, the more effectively he or she will target the cancer itself and protect the normal tissue. But it requires very sharp shooting and very good judgment. A therapist trying to spare normal tissue may confine efforts to a small field. But then he or she runs the risk of leaving some part of the cancer untreated. It is a question of balancing too much against too little, and such balances obviously require the best efforts of the best people.

Even when treatment is perfectly targeted, radiation can cause permanent problems. For one, it can destroy salivary glands throughout the mouth. This leaves the patient with a permanently dry mouth, a condition called *xerostomia*. Xerostomia can subsequently cause infections of the teeth and jaw.

Another serious problem with radiation treatment is that the damage it does to normal tissue is permanent and, indeed, can increase over time. Tissue damaged by radiation is especially vulnerable to infection, which itself may be hard to treat. Thus, insignificant infections that normally would heal without a problem can cause significant damage.

One of the most feared complications that can follow radiation treatment of oral cancer is the infection of the irradiated jawbone. That risk is so common that, before treatment starts, great pains will be taken to eliminate all sources of infection. For some patients, that means full dental extraction before treatment.

A fairly recent development in radiation treatment temporarily implants small radioactive seeds directly into a cancer. This method spares surrounding tissues and allows a high dose of radiation to be targeted to a small area. Such treatment is ideally suited to cancers in the floor of the mouth, but it is available only at major medical centers.

In the case of large lesions of the head and neck, both surgery and radiation will be used. In intermediate and advanced cancers, where, by definition, the cancers are larger and have spread to the neck, the large lymph nodes in the neck must be surgically removed. If the cancer has spread only to the small lymph nodes or if the size of the primary cancer suggests that the cancer has spread, radiation treatment will be used.

Chemotherapy is not a primary treatment for oral cancer, but it *is* used to supplement both radiation and surgery. In the case of radiation, chemotherapy may cut down on the amount of radiation needed, thus reducing its negative effects. Once again, chemotherapy is part of the juggling act your medical team tries to perform. The chemicals, even as they attack the cancer cells, can further weaken your already weakened immune system.

For head and neck cancers, the use of radiation and chemotherapy either before or after surgery is still controversial, and the studies are inconclusive. Indeed, in the case of advanced cancers of this type, there is no one best treatment, and all treatments carry risk. For that reason, we advise that patients get a second opinion. By hearing several physicians discuss various options, the patient will gain clearer understanding of a complex situation.

Cancer is a painful subject, and oral cancer raises especially unpleasant problems. Yet, once again, the bright side is prevention. The best way to avoid oral cancer is to maintain a diet and lifestyle that are good for the body, which means, among other things, good for the immune system.

Even if cancer comes, with proper awareness, the patient can catch these cancers early, when they are most easily and most effectively treatable. Screening for head and neck cancers should be part of your annual checkup, and be included with such other lifesaving exams as a mammogram, Pap smear, PSA, rectal exam, and sigmoidoscopy.

SHAWN TODAY

Shawn knows that it was only by luck that his cancer was diagnosed early and, therefore, that he got early and effective treatments. He's healthy today and intends to remain so. He eats a proper diet, exercises regularly, and, besides carefully monitoring his oral cavity, he gets annual medical checkups.

IN A NUTSHELL

Incidence:

Cancer of the larynx most often appears in people over the age of 55, and men are more likely to get it than women. More African Americans than whites have cancer of the larynx, and more die of it.

Causes:

- Smoking, especially in combination with alcohol
- Chewing tobacco.

Prevention:

- Stop smoking.
- Maintain good oral hygiene.
- Eat a well-balanced diet.

Diagnosis:

Be alert to:

- Nonhealing ulcer in mouth, tongue, lips
- Red or white colored patches in the mouth or on the lips
- A change in the voice, like hoarseness
- A lump or mass in the neck.

Your doctor will:

- Use a flexible or rigid laryngoscope
- Obtain a biopsy sample.

Treatment:

Small early cancers can be treated with surgery alone. Radiation can also be used if the cancer is located on the vocal chords. Larger cancers are treated with surgery and radiation. Chemotherapy, surgery, and radiation are used for larger cancers that have spread to other sites or for cancers of the head and neck that have reoccurred after the initial treatment.

Prognosis:

For small cancers, long-term survival is excellent. Survival is poor for those cancers that have spread to distant sites like the lung. Less then 20 percent of these patients are alive after five years.

NINETEEN

HIV and Cancer

HIV/AIDS

TOM MOORE WAS ONLY THIRTY when it began—night sweats and fever, dramatic weight loss. For a while, he tried to think it was nothing more serious than work pressure that had him down. He'd just been promoted at his ad agency, and though he loved the new job and the new money, he found himself working twice as hard as before. So maybe that was it. But as the weeks went on, he knew in his heart that it was more.

He was suffering headaches so badly he couldn't think, and sometimes, during the day, he fell into a kind of stupor. Increasingly he felt nausea and sometimes he had diarrhea. He was eating less and less, and losing much of what little he did eat. There were lumps at the base of his neck, which, although they didn't hurt, wouldn't go away.

When he at last went to his family doctor, things moved quickly. Then Tom's life came to a terrible halt. After a biopsy and a few other tests, Tom heard the crushing news. He had HIV/AIDS (human immunodeficiency syndrome/acquired immunodeficiency syndrome), and it was complicated by B-cell lymphoma. Despite treatment, Tom was dead six months later.

In the United States, approximately 1 in 50 black men and 1 in 160 black women are infected with HIV.

There's still debate over how long the virus has been active in human beings, but the AIDS epidemic didn't hit the United States until the 1980s. Today, in this country, as in much of the world, it is a plague of terrifying proportions. For African Americans, it is a disaster. We are losing young men and women full of hope and promise to a disease within our power to control. But to do that we must first face the grim facts. Here they are, as the Center for Disease Control (CDC) in Atlanta has gathered them:

- As of 2004, 50 percent of all newly diagnosed AIDS cases were among African Americans.
- In 2002, HIV/AIDS was reported to be the second leading cause of death for African Americans between the ages of thirty-five to forty-four.
- In 2004, 50 percent of all new HIV/AIDS diagnoses were African-Americans even though they make up only about 13 percent of the U.S. population.

Keep in mind that these figures represent only the reported cases and that this epidemic hasn't yet peaked, and you will see the scope of the disaster.

AIDS itself is an active disease of the immune system. HIV is a virus. It causes AIDS. Most people don't develop symptoms of AIDS for about ten years after they've become HIV-positive.

HOW THE HIV/AIDS TREND CAN BE CHANGED

The Centers for Disease Control is making a most vigorous effort to fight the spread of the HIV epidemic in the black community. CDC programs are directed at risk-reduction counseling, case management services, community outreach, and providing access to HIV testing and treatment. The CDC also assists national and community-based organizations, including churches, to build the structures they need to carry out these same services. The services funded by the CDC through the churches include programs designed to study risk behaviors in injection-drug users, and among gay and bisexual black men.

Because of the terrible toll HIV/AIDS has taken of black women, and, through them, of infants who come into the world infected with the virus, organizations such as the CDC, the Black AIDS Institute, and Sister Love, Inc. and Balm in Gilead are promoting AIDS awareness in women as well the use of condoms and other preventive techniques.

For these programs to work, they need active participation by churches and other black organizations. If the African-American community is to preserve itself, we must all take it upon ourselves to work for the caging of this dread disease that has already caused so much damage. Though this is everybody's job—the lawyer and the professor, the worker and the professional, the prisoner and the homeless person, the housewife and the woman in the street—we think that the churches must take the lead.

To have awareness means we must know what AIDS is, how we get it, what it does to us, and even, in the worst case, how we can live with it. It means we must use condoms. Finally, it means getting tested if there is any possibility that we have been infected.

How, after all, *can* we control the disease when people who may be infected refuse to be tested? Like a refusal to wear a condom, fear of testing is reckless, even suicidal. It expresses disregard for other people's lives and for our own life. We all know the strength of sexual desire, but we should know that it has to be weighed against other values. When people are willing to risk their own lives and the lives of those they have taken as lovers in order to sustain their pleasure, something is seriously amiss.

We are all too good to die of AIDS. We are all too smart not to see the silliness of trading one's life for the "freedom" of not wearing a condom.

WHAT IS HIV/AIDS?

AIDS was first identified in the United States in 1981, when significant numbers of people were discovered to suffer from pneumonia and from a kind of tumor called Kaposi's sarcoma. Unexplained immune dysfunction began showing up in doctors' offices.

The wide occurrence of this syndrome among homosexual men and injection-drug users led researchers to see that the disease was infectious. That suspicion was tragically confirmed when there occurred an outbreak of AIDS among hemophiliacs, who had contracted it through blood transfusions. In 1984, the HIV virus itself was identified as the cause of the AIDS crisis.

WHAT ARE THE SYMPTOMS?

AIDS can strike anywhere in the body, damaging virtually any organ or tissue. Once the disease has weakened your immune system, the door is open to other diseases. In general, the lungs, the gastrointestinal tract, the nervous system, and the skin are areas most likely to be involved.

HOW HIV IS TRANSMITTED

HIV is transmitted in three ways:

- Unprotected sexual contact—both vaginal and semenal secretions can carry HIV

- Blood and blood products
- Transmission from infected mothers to their offspring.

Transmission Through Sexual Contact

The most common means of transmission are sexual contact and contaminated blood. In studies of homosexual men, the incidence of HIV infections increased with the number of sexual partners, and with the practice of anal intercourse or other practices that lead to trauma of skin or mucous membranes.

> *The most common means of transmission are sexual contact and contaminated blood.*

AIDS is *not* a disease that only homosexuals can get. Although in this country transmission is less common between male and female sex partners, throughout the third world, where the incidence of AIDS infection is rising at a terrifying pace, the disease is spread mainly through heterosexual vaginal intercourse.

AIDS can live in the body for ten years and even longer without causing severe symptoms. This means that many people infected with AIDS don't know it, and their lovers have no way of knowing either. It is all too easy for us to be infected or to infect someone else without knowing it.

At the same time, it is just as easy to prevent such infection from taking place. Get tested and be sure that your lover or lovers have been tested, too. At the very least, unless you are certain that you and your partner are *not* infected, use condoms. A latex condom is one of several barriers—latex gloves for health workers, plastic wrap, and dental dams also work—known to stop AIDS. (Diaphragms do *not* offer protection because the virus can enter at any part of the vagina.)

> *The proper use of condoms can decrease HIV transmission by 90 percent.*

The proper use of condoms can decrease HIV transmission by 90 percent. Nothing could be more terrible than that fact. What it suggests—this is worth repeating—is that hundreds of thousands of people are contracting a deadly disease simply because they are too thoughtless to protect themselves with condoms. Surely human life is meant for some higher purpose than to be thrown away.

Transmission Through the Blood

Transmission of AIDS through the blood occurs when intravenous drug users exchange contaminated needles. Two ways to control AIDS, then, are to provide drug abuse treatment and counseling, and to make sterile needles available. Blood transfusions were once a major source of infection, but they aren't any longer because donors are screened for the virus.

Health care workers are also at risk when working with infected patients. They have learned to take great care. Getting infected by accidental sticks with contaminated needles or other medical instruments happens—though fortunately not often.

Transmission from Infected Mothers

The transmission of HIV from an infected mother to her infant during pregnancy, delivery, or breast-feeding, is a terrible problem. What could be worse than the transmission of death through the very processes of life? New drugs offer new hope in the control of this transmission. Yet in this country, and on a world-scale, transmission of HIV from an infected mother is one of the most overwhelming and immediate problems our species faces.

HOW YOU CAN'T GET HIV

In 2005, the National Institutes of Health's Division of Allergy and Infectious Diseases listed these ways that you *cannot* get HIV:

- Not by sitting on a toilet seat.
- Not by eating food prepared by someone who has the virus.

- Not by holding, hugging, or touching someone who has the virus.
- Not from swimming in a pool with someone who has the virus.
- Not from working with or attending school with someone who has the virus.
- Not from a mosquito bite.
- Probably not from the tears, saliva, urine, and feces of someone who has the virus. Small amounts of virus have been found in these excretions, but the concentration is almost certainly too low to cause infection.

PREVENTION

Except for the infants who are born with it, nobody has to get AIDS. Avoiding it means, simply, living responsibly.

AIDS can be prevented in any one of the following ways, depending on circumstance:

- Abstinence, obviously, is the surest way. A serious case for abstinence can be made when the alternative may be death. But it's also true, as Dr. Elders argues, that abstinence is a difficult choice.
- Monogamous sex with a partner one knows is AIDS free. This is a path we think closer to ordinary human capacity. People need to understand that to have intercourse with strangers who may be infected with HIV, and to do so without the use of condoms, is to play Russian roulette.
- Wear a condom if, after reading this far, you choose to continue to make love to many partners. Not wearing a condom is to risk suicide. Choose to live. Wear a condom.
- Use sterile needles if you're a drug user. Short of kicking the habit, the best thing you can do for yourself is to make sure that you're using sterile needles.
- Avoid behavior that promotes HIV. Think how much you could be risking.

DIAGNOSIS

Doctors have several resources in diagnosing HIV/AIDS:

- The patient's own history of intravenous drug use or of unprotected sex
- The patient's symptoms, which, though not specific, may include fever, night sweats, loss of weight, and painless enlargement of the lymph nodes
- Western blot, a molecular biological screening test that examines viral proteins
- A test that evaluates CD4 , a type of lymphocyte that is crucial to the immune process
- A test that measures the HIV viral load and thus helps measure the effectiveness of treatment.

Other tests continue to be developed and tested.

CANCER AND HIV

One of the many unpleasant diseases that can develop from an active AIDS infection is non-Hodgkin's lymphoma. AIDS patients have a sixty times greater risk for this disease than people without AIDS. This is because AIDS attacks the lymph system generally and the CD4 lymphocyte particularly. This means that it attacks the systemic processes with which the body fights infection.

Treating AIDS can be a medical nightmare. Often it means treating not simply the primary infection but also major secondary ones like cancer and pneumonia.

THE IMMUNE SYSTEM AND AIDS

Your body's system for fighting infection and resisting the development of cancer is called the lymphatic system. There's a lot about it we don't understand, but this much we *do* know. White blood cells called *lymphocytes* are carried through the channels of your lymphatic system, in a clear and virtually colorless liquid called *lymph*. These, lymphocytes, with the help of other disease-fighting cells, cleanse the body of toxins, bacteria, viruses, and cancer cells. Without a working immune system our bodies would soon be overwhelmed with bacterial or viral infections, or with cancer.

HIV destroys the immune system by inactivating lymphocytes or making them less effective in fighting bacteria, viruses, and cancer. The end result is overwhelming infection and cancers like lymphoma.

There are essentially two kinds of lymphoma, Hodgkin's and non-Hodgkin's. The resemblance and difference between them isn't essential here, except to say that the non-Hodgkin's lymphoma is emerging as a typical sign of HIV infection. Non-Hodgkin's lymphoma is commonly known as B-cell lymphoma. The B-cells that multiply in this disease are caused by genetic changes that allow them to convert into malignant ones.

AIDS patients have a 57 percent greater risk for non-Hodgkin's lymphoma than do people without AIDS.

DOES AIDS CAUSE NON-HODGKIN'S LYMPHOMA?

The truth is that we don't know if AIDS causes non-Hodgkin's lymphoma. Some experts believe that AIDS is not a direct cause but rather provides a permissive environment in which lymphoma develops.

TREATMENT

If non-Hodgkin's lymphoma does occur, treatment is difficult and the prognosis poor. Keep in mind that the body's immune system is already compromised by the HIV infection. It is further weakened by the chemical agents needed to treat the lymphoma, which are likely to cause bone marrow suppression and thus weaken the immune system. In this way, AIDS patients can succumb to relatively mild diseases like pharyngitis.

Because the treatment of HIV must be given along with therapy for the lymphoma, prognosis is very poor. Patients with AIDS-related B-cell lymphoma rarely live more than nine months from the time they were first diagnosed with AIDS.

AIDS patients do have choices in their treatment. Before we get into the specifics of treatment, we need to stress that the best way to live with AIDS—as odd as this may sound— is to stay as well as one can physically and emotionally:

- Take special care with all matters of personal hygiene.
- Also, avoid unnecessary exposure to potential infection.

  Avoid weakening the immune system, which means:

- Don't smoke. Smoking damages the immune system.
- Avoid stress. Stress weakens the immune system.
- Drink little or no alcohol. Alcohol weakens the immune system.
- Avoid using street drugs. They will only weaken you faster.

The patient who wants to live with AIDS rather than die of it must in some cases change his or her lifestyle. But by making such changes, the patient will also be choosing to control the disease, instead of waiting passively for the outcome. Our chapter on "Living with Cancer" sketches some of the resources the AIDS patient will need to manage the disease with as little stress as possible. We don't claim that it's easy to be ill with a life-threatening disease and to remain calm in the process. We say only that there are better and worse ways to shoot for that goal.

MEDICAL TREATMENT FOR HIV/AIDS

Living with AIDS: A Guide for African Americans (Hilton Publishing, Chicago, IL, 2006) specifies the different medications usually prescribed to fight AIDS. These include:

Nucleoside Transciptase Inhibitors (nukes)

These drugs prevent the viral RNA from changing into DNA, by the use of an enzyme found in the cytoplasm of your host cells called "reverse transcriptase enzyme." These drugs all have been associated with the development of a condition called lactic acidosis and severe liver problems, which are relatively rare but serious side effects. Specific drugs will have specific additional side effects. These drugs include:

- Abacavir (Ziagen; Trizivir): About 5 percent of patients will have a serious allergic reaction that may cause death if the drug is not stopped right away. Signs of this serious reaction include a skin rash or one or more of these symptoms: fever, nausea, vomiting, diarrhea, abdominal (stomach) pain, extreme tiredness, achiness, generally ill feeling, sore throat, shortness of breath, cough.

    Other side effects with Abacavir are nausea, vomiting, feeling generally ill or tired, headache, diarrhea, loss of appetite and changes in body fat.

- Didanosine (DDI) may cause peripheral neuropathy (a problem with the nerves in your hands or feet), inflamed pancreas, a serious side effect, and changes in vision. Other side effects with DDI are diarrhea, neuropathy, chills or fever, rash, abdominal pain, weakness, headache and nausea and vomiting.

- Lamivudine (3TC; Epivir): Children with a history of prior antiretroviral nucleoside exposure, pancreatitis or other significant risk factors for the development of pancreatitis should use this medication with caution. Fat redistribution may also occur.

    Other adverse reactions may include nausea and vomiting, diarrhea, anorexia and/or decreased appetite, stomach upset (pain, cramp and indigestion), dizziness, fatigue and/ or malaise, headache, fever or chills, dreams, insomnia and other sleep disorders, skin rash, problems with nerves, depression, cough, nasal problems, muscle pain and joint pain.

- Stavudine (D4T; Zerit) may cause nerve damage of the hands and feet (peripheral neuropathy), and pancreatitis (inflammation of the pancreas, which may result in stomach pain, nausea or vomiting). Other side effects may include headache, diarrhea, rash, nausea and vomiting, stomach pain, muscle pain, insomnia, loss of appetite, chills or fever, allergic reactions and blood disorders.
- Trizivir is a combination of AZT, 3TC and Abacavir. See each drug for side effect profile. Trizivir can also cause dizziness and pain or tingling in your hands or feet.
- Zalcitabine (DDC; Hivid) may cause severe peripheral neuropathy (tingling in arms and legs), particularly in those patients with advanced cases of the disease. It may also cause pancreatitis and hepatic failure (which may be fatal). Other serious side effects may include oral ulcers, stomach ulcers, heart failure, changes in body fat, and allergic reaction.
- Zidovudine (Retrovir, previously known as AZT), may cause bone marrow suppression, blood disorders (severe anemia and low levels of blood cells) and muscle weakness. Other side effects may include nausea, vomiting, weakness, headache, generally feeling ill, anorexia, constipation, stomach upset (pain, cramp and indigestion), joint pain, chills, feeling tired, elevated liver enzymes, trouble sleeping, muscle and joint pain and neuropathy (nervous system disorder).

Nucleotide Reverse Transcriptase Inhibitors

- Tenofovir (Viread) may cause diarrhea, nausea, vomiting and intestinal gas. Other less common side effects may include weakness, inflammation of the pancreas, low blood phosphate, dizziness, shortness of breath and rash. Some patients have developed kidney problems. In some cases of patients taking anti-HIV medicine, body fat changes have also been seen.

Non-nucleoside Transcriptase Inhibitors (NNRTIs)
These drugs work in a way similar to nukes above. NNRTIs include:

- Delavirdine mesylate (Rescriptor) may cause a skin rash on the upper body and upper arms, sometimes on the neck and face. The rash usually appears as a red area on the skin with slight bumps; it may be itchy. Other side effects may include headache, nausea, diarrhea and tiredness.
- Efavirenz (Stocrin; Sustiva): A small number of patients experience severe depression, strange thoughts, angry behavior, thoughts of suicide and, very rarely, actual suicide. Other side effects include dizziness, trouble sleeping, drowsiness, trouble concentrating and/or unusual dreams, rash, tiredness, upset stomach, vomiting and diarrhea and changes in body fat.
- Nevirapine (Viramune) may cause a severe rash and hepatitis. In rare cases, liver problems may lead to liver failure, which can lead to liver transplants or death. Other side effects include changes in body fat.

Protease Inhibitors
Protease inhibitors are very powerful in killing the virus in combination with NRT and NNRTIs. They work by blocking the enzyme protease, which is used to assemble the virus in the cytoplasm of the host cell. All the protease inhibitors have been associated with increased bleeding in patients with hemophilia, GI intolerance, elevated glucose and increases in cholesterol, triglycerides and body fat redistribution.

These drugs, with their side effects, include:

- Amprenavir (Agenerase) may cause a severe rash. Other side effects may include diarrhea, nausea and vomiting, a tingling feeling, especially around the mouth, and change in taste. These effects are usually mild to moderate. Other reported side effects include depression and mood problems, changes in body fat, seizures, drowsiness, fast heart rate and kidney and blood abnormalities. Other side effects may include high blood sugar or diabetes, diabetes complications, high cholesterol or high triglycerides.

- Indinavir (Crixivan): Some patients treated with Crixivan developed kidney stones. In some of these patients, development of kidney stones leads to more severe kidney problems, including kidney failure or inflammation of the kidneys, or kidney infection that sometimes spreads to the blood.

   Some patients treated with Crixivan have had rapid breakdown of red blood cells (hemolytic anemia) which in some cases was severe or resulted in death. Some patients treated with Crixivan also have had liver problems including liver failure and death.

   Other side effects include diabetes and high blood sugar, increased bleeding in patients with hemophilia, severe muscle pain and weakness, changes in body fat, increased liver enzymes, abdominal pain, fatigue or weakness, low red blood cell count, flank pain, painful urination, feeling unwell, nausea, upset stomach, diarrhea, vomiting, acid regurgitation, increased or decreased appetite, back pain, headache, dizziness, taste changes, rash, itchy skin, yellowing of the skin and/or eyes, upper respiratory infection, dry skin, sore throat, swollen kidneys due to blocked urine, allergic reactions, severe skin reactions, heart problems including heart attack, stroke, abdominal swelling, indigestion, inflammation of the kidneys, inflammation of the pancreas, joint pain, depression, itching, hives, change in skin color, hair loss, ingrown toenails with or without infection, crystals in the urine and numbness of the mouth.

- Lopinavir/ritonavir (Kaletra) is a combination of Lopinavir and ritonavir. The most commonly reported side effects are abdominal pain, abnormal bowel movements, diarrhea, feeling weak and/or tired, headache and nausea.

   Children taking Kaletra may sometimes get a skin rash. Liver problems, sometimes severe, may occur in patients, as may pancreatitis, which may also be severe. Some patients have large increases in triglycerides and cholesterol. Diabetes and high blood sugar may occur in patients taking protease inhibitors such as Kaletra. Changes in body fat have also been seen in some patients taking antiretroviral therapy. And some patients with hemophilia have increased bleeding with protease inhibitors.

- Nelfinavir mesylate (Viracept). The most common side effect is diarrhea. Other side effects include nausea, gas and rash. Diabetes and high blood sugar (hyperglycemia) may also occur. Changes in body fat in patients taking antiretroviral therapy may occur. Some patients with hemophilia may have increased bleeding with protease inhibitors.

- Ritonavir (Norvir). Side effects include feeling weak/tired, nausea, vomiting, loss of appetite, abdominal pain, changes in taste, numbness and tingling of the hands or feet or around the lips, headache and dizziness. Liver problems, sometimes severe, may occur in patients, as may pancreatitis, which may also be severe. Some patients have large increases in triglycerides and cholesterol. Diabetes and high blood sugar may also occur. Allergic reactions can range from mild to severe. Some patients with hemophilia may have increased bleeding with protease inhibitors. Some patients taking anti-HIV medicines may also have changes in body fat.

- Saquinavir (Invirase) (hard gel form), or Fortovase (soft gel) may cause diarrhea, nausea, abdominal discomfort and heartburn. Other side effects include abdominal pain, gas, vomiting, fatigue, headache, body aches, anxiety, depression, warts, change in sexual appetite, taste changes, constipation, sleeplessness, weight gain, gum disease, numbness or tingling, fever, convulsions, itching and rash, shortness of breath, fungal infection, hepatitis, night sweats, blurred vision, difficult urination, dizziness, coughing blood, bleeding in the brain, ulcers, inflamed pancreas and rapid heart rate. Also reported are

increases in liver function tests, increased blood sugar levels
and changes in body fat.

Fusion Inhibitors

Fusion inhibitors, one of the newest treatments for HIV, prevent the
attachment of the virus to the CD4 receptor on the cell surface. In
short, they block HIV's ability to infect healthy CD4 cells. They are
to be used only with other anti-HIV medicines.

- Enfuvirtide (Fuzeon): Because enfuvirtide is injected, it can
  cause injection-site reactions, including itching, swelling, red-
  ness, pain or tenderness, hardened skin and bumps. Other side
  effects may include bacterial pneumonia, serious allergic reactions such as trouble breathing, fever with vomiting, skin rash,
  blood in the urine and swelling of the feet. Call your health
  care provider immediately if these reactions occur. Still other
  side effects, in combination with other anti-HIV medicines,
  may include pain and numbness in feet or legs, loss of sleep,
  depression, weakness or loss of strength, muscle pain,
  decreased appetite, constipation and pancreas problems.

With the help of these antiviral drugs, we can reduce AIDS to a
manageable, long-term illness. Keep in mind, however, that these
drugs are very expensive. Some of the newest and most effective can
cost as much as $16,000 a year.

A second family of medicines used in the war against AIDS is
used *prophylactically*—that is, they help the body defend against
specific diseases. Antibiotics help ward off a devastating pneumonia.
Other drugs help ward off tuberculosis and other infections that
might otherwise take advantage of the body's weakened immune
system. Kaposi's sarcoma can also be treated by a variety of drugs,
either singly or in combination. X-ray therapy may also be helpful.
For those who can afford to use them, many of these drugs can also
create problems. There can be severe side effects, including some
life-threatening ones.

KAPOSI'S SARCOMA

Kaposi's sarcoma (KS) can occur in non-AIDS patients. It was first described as a disease found in the extremities of elderly men. Since then, in Africa, a more aggressive form involves the internal organs and lymph nodes. Still another form may occur in patients who receive immunosuppressive therapy—for kidney and liver transplants, for example. In these cases, tumors often subside or even vanish when the immunosuppression is stopped. This strengthened the view that the development of Karposi's sarcoma is the sign of a weakened and incompetent immune system.

TREATMENT OF KAPOSI'S SARCOMA

As in the treatment of B-cell lymphoma, treatment of KS is difficult because the chemical agents or x-ray treatment used to reduce the malignancy may further weaken the immune system and aggravate the primary condition—AIDS.

Cryotherapy (which freezes the tumor), injected drugs like interferon alpha, and x-ray treatment may also be used to treat individual tumors. Systemic treatment involves alpha-interferon, doxorubicin, vincristine, or AZT, given singly or in combination. These drugs are injected in the vein and reach all the diseased areas. The patient's response to these drugs must be carefully monitored. Alpha-interferon can cause flulike symptoms and may be tolerated only for a brief period.

OTHER CANCERS RELATED TO AIDS

Other cancers occur frequently in HIV/AIDS patients. *Papillomavirus* infections, which can cause small, benign tumors in the breast, intestine, mucus membrane, or skin, occur frequently among these patients, and can develop into more serious cancers—such as uterine cervical cancer and anal cancer.

A test to detect the human papilloma virus (HPV) should be done in HIV patients because they are susceptible to this virus. Treatment of premalignant lesions will prevent the formation of cervical and anal cancers.

Squamous cell cancers of the mouth, tongue, larynx, and esophagus also appear to have a higher rate of incidence and a more rapidly increased rate of incidence in HIV patients than in the general population.

IN A NUTSHELL

Incidence:
- African Americans make up 50 percent of all AIDS cases.
- In the U.S., the estimated number of diagnosed AIDS cases through 2003 is 929,985.
- African Americans make up 12.3 percent of the population but 50 percent of all cases.
- By the end of 2004, 201,045 African Americans had died of AIDS.
- Of all the races in America, African Americans have the lowest survival rate for HIV/AIDS.
- In 2004, the rate of AIDS diagnoses for African-American women was nineteen times higher than the rate for whites.
- During the same period, the rate of HIV infection for African-American men was eight times higher than that of white men.

Cause:
A virus (HIV) that is transmitted to humans from another human through blood or semen. It can pass from a pregnant mother to the fetus.

Risk factors:
- Unprotected sex
- Multiple sex partners
- Anal intercourse

- Contaminated needles for intravenous injection, especially when needles are shared for addictive drugs.

Prevention:
- Avoid risk factors
- Use condoms.

Diagnosis:
Be alert to:
- Weight loss
- Recurrent lung infections or pneumonia
- Progressive weight loss
- Swollen lymph nodes
- Deterioration of the immune system.

Treatment:
Multiple drugs must be used, including antiviral medications and antibiotics to treat frequent infections. Patient must be monitored closely to assure that the virus is being adequately controlled.

There currently is no cure once infected with HIV. Life can be significantly prolonged through strict adherence to treatment programs.

TWENTY

Cancers of Lower Incidence

I N THIS CHAPTER, I will describe cancers that occur at a relatively low rate among blacks. But cancer is cancer. If I am the only one among millions unfortunate enough to be affected, the incidence is 100 percent in me. The hard fact is that I have two or more close friends infected with each of the cancers I have described in this chapter—except cancer of the penis.

HODGKIN'S DISEASE

Hodgkin's disease (HD) is a cancerous disease of the lymphatic system that primarily involves the lymph nodes. It is less common in blacks than in whites.

Hodgkin's can strike with relatively few symptoms in the early stages. When there *are* early symptoms, they often come as a triad (in threes):

- Fever
- Drenching night sweats
- Weight loss.

Diagnosis

Diagnosis is made when, after enlarged lymph nodes have been detected, biopsy reveals malignant cells typical of HD. Staging is then determined according to which lymph nodes and groups of lymph nodes are involved. The nodes can be in the neck, chest, or groin area.

Physical examination and CT scans of chest and abdomen are part of the diagnostic process. Surgical exploration of the abdomen may be necessary to determine whether lymph nodes below the diaphragm, or in the spleen or liver, are involved.

In the majority of cases (some 80 percent), involvement is limited to areas *above* the diaphragm, especially the anterior upper chest (mediastinum).

Treatment

Treatment is usually by radiation or chemotherapy. The latter is commonly a drug combination called MOPP or ABVD.

Successful treatment of HD can sometimes be followed by the occurrence of other tumors in the lungs, breast, stomach, or by leukemia. Tobacco use, of course, heightens the risk that lung cancer will develop after the HD has been successfully treated. HD patients must be followed for the rest of their lives.

Prognosis

Appropriately treated, 80 percent of the people with stage I or II Hodgkin's disease survive for at least ten years. In cases where the disease is already widespread, the five-year survival rate is 60 percent.

LEUKEMIA

Leukemia is cancer of the bone marrow cells. Because, like lymphoma, leukemia is involved with the immune system, it arises from any of the many cell types that make up the immune system.

Leukemias can be acute or chronic, depending on the intensity and the suddenness of symptoms and the particular cell type. Acute leukemia can strike suddenly and in a deadly fashion. A bridge partner of mine fainted suddenly during a game, without previous symptoms. Though he was revived, he developed a high fever and died within twenty-four hours, despite heroic medical efforts. He never knew he had leukemia.

Chronic leukemia is less sudden in onset and severity, and moves more slowly.

How the Disease Works

The specific cause of leukemia is unknown, but we know something about what happens once the disease is established. An unknown bodily event triggers a mechanism whereby young blood cells of a specific type remain immature and proliferate (divide and multiply) rapidly. Both genetic and viral causes can lead to these changes.

These immature cells choke out the healthy cells of the bone marrow that protect against infection and bleeding. Bleeding and infection are usually early symptoms of leukemia, but they don't always appear early, and diagnosis does not depend on their presence.

Diagnosis

Diagnosis begins with symptoms: anemia (low blood count) and infection. Blood tests will provide a presumptive diagnosis. A final diagnosis will depend on biopsy of the bone marrow—usually from a bone near the hip or from the sternum. If the disease is present, the biopsy will reveal the characteristic immature cells.

Treatment of leukemia can be effective. Chemotherapy can bring about periods when all signs of the disease temporarily vanish (remissions) and sometimes cure. But remission and cure are most likely when the disease is caught early and treated effectively. Bone marrow transplants are sometimes an effective treatment for leukemia, and a blood cell (platelet) transfusion can protect against bleeding.

One kind of leukemia, chronic myelogenous leukemia, has been identified as having a genetic cause. In this form of leukemia, a so-called Philadelphia chromosome is present in the bone marrow cells.

Prognosis for Leukemia

The prognosis for leukemia is guarded. When acute leukemia is diagnosed early and treated effectively, remissions and cures are possible. But many die early of this disease.

In chronic leukemia, the prognosis is somewhat better. With treatment, many patients survive for three or four years, and others go on to live longer and productive lives.

CANCER OF THE TESTICLE

Between 6,000 and 8,000 men are diagnosed with testicular cancers each year. Although it accounts for only 1 percent of all cancers in men, in young men fifteen to forty years old, it is the most common form of cancer. It may also occur in young boys, but such cases make up only 3 percent of all testicular cancer cases. African Americans are five times less likely than whites to get testicular cancer, and while the rate of this cancer has doubled among white Americans, it has remained the same for African Americans. White American men have about five times the risk of African-American men and more than twice the risk of Asian-American men. The risk for testicular cancer has doubled among white Americans in the past forty years but has remained the same for African Americans. No one knows why.

Causes of Testicular Cancer

Although we don't know the causes of testicular cancer, we do know that it occurs more often in undescended testicles. This means that the testicle remains high in the scrotum or is even hidden in the back of the abdomen; it is not hanging low in the scrotum.

If you can't feel your testicle in the scrotum, have it checked out. You may decide that you want it repaired, which can be done through surgery.

Most Scrotal Masses Aren't Cancers

The fact is most scrotal masses *aren't* cancers. The most common masses are *hydrocele* (water in the scrotal sac) and *hernia*. Hernia is easily diagnosed by physical examination. Hydrocele is diagnosed by simply placing a light behind the scrotum. If there is water in the sac, it will transilluminate—that is, light will pass through it. It can be treated surgically in severe cases.

Let your doctor decide what the mass is. If you discover a non-tender, solid mass, it needs to be examined. If the doctor eliminates hydrocele and hernia, he or she will want to have the mass biopsied. If the biopsy result is positive, the prognosis will depend on the stage of the cancer. Most cancers of this type are highly curable if detected early. Treatment usually means removal of the diseased testicle, followed by chemotherapy. Happily, one testicle can do the work of two.

Here are the key facts about testicular cancer:

- Blacks are less likely than whites to develop cancer of the testicle.
- Most lumps in the scrotum aren't cancerous.
- If you feel an enlargement or mass in your scrotum, don't procrastinate. See your doctor.
- If your child doesn't have a full scrotum and the testicle isn't "down," see your doctor about having it brought down. Doing this will help prevent a cancer of the testicle from forming. Having the operation done by the age of five or six guarantees the best success, and removes this important risk factor for testicular cancer.

CARCINOMA OF THE PENIS

Carcinoma of the penis is very rare, but it happens. The four cases I've seen were all white men, among whom the disease is more common. But because this cancer is so easily detected, you should know the signs.

This cancer *presents* (makes itself known) as a sore on the penis's foreskin that does not heal. The sore is usually painless unless a secondary infection sets in. Carcinoma of the penis is more common in uncircumcised males.

Cancer is not the only possible cause of sores on the penis. Sexually transmitted diseases can produce the same symptom.

If you have a sore on the penis, don't hesitate to get it examined and treated. Carcinoma of the penis can be treated if it's caught early.

BREAST CANCER IN THE MALE

Breast cancer can occur in the male although it is rare. One percent of all breast cancers occur in men. This cancer occurs in males with high estrogen levels. Alcohol damage to the liver is a cause of such high levels.

Stage for stage, survival rates for men are similar to those of women. But in the case of men, presumably because this isn't a condition men look for, diagnosis often comes later.

Cancer presents in the male breast just as it does in the female: through a lump or through a roughening or rash on the skin around the nipple.

Treatment for this form of cancer is usually in the form of modified radical mastectomy, usually with a skin graft. Irradiation and chemotherapy may be used selectively.

MULTIPLE MYELOMA

Although this cancer accounts for only 1 percent of all cancers, it occurs twice as frequently in blacks than in whites. We don't know why it starts, but it starts with an overactive production of cells in the bone marrow known as *plasma cells*. Eventually, that overproduction will cause erosion of nearby bone, thus leading to pain and fractures.

Symptoms include:

- Anemia
- Weakness
- Fever.

Bone defects will show on x-rays. The kidney and liver may be involved.

Chemotherapy using prednisone is the preferred therapy. Bone marrow transplantation is sometimes used, but with caution.

Untreated, patients with multiple myeloma rarely survive more than six months. With treatment, survival is two and a half years.

PART III

Human Questions

TWENTY-ONE

Equality in Health Care?

ACCESS

MARY DEBOSE WAS FRIGHTENED when she saw bright red blood in her stools, but the doctor in her local emergency room reassured her. That he reassured her without having done his job thoroughly didn't occur to Mary. She assumed that doctors knew their business and did it well.

Mary's doctor *did* examine her. One glance at her anus showed that she had a few hemorrhoids. Without looking any further, he told her to get an over-the-counter medication and use it—and that was that.

But for Mary, as it turned out, that *wasn't* that. She used the prescribed suppositories, but the bleeding continued. Mary thought about returning to the hospital, but the doctor had made her uncomfortable, calling her by her first name as if she were a child, and talking to her as if she didn't have any sense. For Mary it felt like the low-grade racism she'd run into often enough in her lifetime not to want any more. Besides, now she knew the cause of the bleeding: it was only hemorrhoids, wasn't it?

Doing the wash one day, Mary's daughter Angie saw blood on her mother's underwear and was frightened. "Mama," she said, "you're going to the doctor. I don't care what you say." Angie made an appointment for her mother with Dr. Scott, whom one of her friends recommended as a good doctor and a careful and kind man. During the physical exam, Dr. Scott saw, just as the emergency ward doctor saw, that Mary had hemorrhoids. But when he took the next diagnostic step of probing her rectum with a gloved finger he felt a firm mass high up.

"Mrs. Debose," he said, "I want you to see a gastroenterologist. He's a doctor who specializes in the digestive system. He'll want to take a sample of that lump and look at the cells. That's the only way we can tell for sure what it is."

The biopsy taken by the gastroenterologist showed that the lump was cancer. During the surgery that followed, it was clear that lymph nodes were involved. Mary came out of the surgery well and responded nicely to the therapy that followed. But her prognosis is guarded. A stage III cancer like hers tends to recur, and her doctors are keeping a careful eye on it.

During one of their talks, Dr. Scott let Mary know that she'd have been in a much better position if the cancer had been diagnosed earlier. She told him why it hadn't. Dr. Scott could only nod his head sadly, wondering to himself whether it was Mary's blackness or the incompetence of the ER doctor that had led to the careless diagnosis.

What should have happened during that first visit Dr. Scott knew very well. Another of his patients, Carol Ingram, had also gone first to the emergency room when she discovered blood in her stool. As in Mary's case, the ER doctor noted a few hemorrhoids right off. But he didn't stop there. He did a rectal, and when he didn't feel a mass, he didn't stop there either. Instead, he sent her to a specialist who, during a lighted exam of her lower bowel (sigmoidoscopy), found a tumor. Biopsy proved that it was cancer.

Carol had surgery. No lymph nodes were involved, and her prognosis is good. Carol happens to be white.

INJUSTICE AND JUSTICE IN THE HEALTH CARE SYSTEM

It's a sad fact that if Dr. Martin Luther King, Jr., were still alive, he would still have to say the same thing about the American health system. What he *did* say was this: "Of all forms of inequality, injustice in health is the most shocking and inhumane." We'll begin by giving you some basic facts about health disparities. Government statistics indicate that while roughly 36% of whites reported themselves in excellent health, for African Americans the number is a little over 29%. Of people who reported themselves in very good health, 32% were whites, and about 28% were African Americans. These disparities hold true at all levels of health: whites are healthier than African Americans and far less likely to fall into poor health. Of those in poor health, the disparities still hold: for whites, 2.1% and for African Americans, 3.6%—or you can say one White person in five is in poor health, compared to one in three African Americans in poor health. Roughly 44% of whites have private medical insurance, against 33.7% of African Americans; and while 12.3% of whites depend on Medicare and Medicaid for health service, 12.7% percent of African Americans do.

"Of all forms of inequality, injustice in health is the most shocking and inhumane."

In most cases, uninsured people have few options when they get sick or injured. They must go to hospital emergency rooms (ERs) for diagnosis and treatment. However dedicated the health providers in ERs may be, emergency rooms are usually crowded, so medical service must be rushed.

Part of the health crisis among African Americans is economic.

DISPARITY

When African Americans do get to doctors, they aren't always treated with the same care and patience as whites. There's something at work here beyond economic discrimination. The American Medical Association (*JAMA*, May 2, 1990) reports that even when blacks gain access to the health care system they're less likely than whites "to receive certain surgical and other therapies." This means that even in a doctor's examination room they may be diagnosed, like Mary Debose, with an illness less serious than they really have, and hustled away with treatment less effective than the treatment they need.

In many cases, the only available medical treatment is the emergency room.

One way this can be corrected is in the medical schools and other schools that train health professionals. We need more black doctors, nurses, nurse practitioners, and physician's assistants, and we need strong programs to ensure an adequate supply of these well-trained professionals. Until that improvement is accomplished, your doctor is likely to be a white male, and doctors, like many other white males, need better awareness of, and sensitivity toward, diversity issues.

When African Americans do get to doctors, they aren't always treated with the same care and patience as whites.

Programs to make that happen have been launched here and there. Dr. Patricia Keener, Chief of Pediatrics at Wishard Hospital in Indianapolis, for example, developed a diversity program for medical students that worked very well. In discussion with African-American community leaders, young doctors in the program learned, for example, that black women didn't like being called by their first names by people they didn't know very well. White doctors might do so in an attempt to be informal and friendly, but the black women resented the practice. Sometimes that resentment translated into not taking prescribed medication, not following recommended diets, or not keeping the next appointment. To correct this, some doctors simply have to become more diplomatic so that they may better be able to treat *all* of their patients. These doctors must sensitize themselves to different customs—whether the patient be black, Asian, Latino, or European.

Prejudice exists in the medical system, and some of it shows itself in ways much worse than the inappropriate use of first names. Disparities in treatment exist, and if you're poor and uninsured, you're not likely to get the kind of care you'd expect if you weren't.

These are serious problems, and we should turn to our politicians to help remedy them. We should turn also to our community leaders to put them in the forefront of issues that need to be addressed locally. And we should do what we can to encourage our young people to enter the medical profession.

But I'm a doctor, not a politician. I know there are some circumstances beyond my personal power to change. I know that I, like other doctors, can sometimes be careless even in matters that I *could* change. The medical system today is driven by profit, and profit means speed. Sometimes doctors don't take the time to explain things as clearly as they should. (Patients say far more than "sometimes." A poll in *Medical Advertising News* found that 90 percent of patients have trouble understanding what their doctors are saying.)

But part of the problem is also in your own hands as a patient.

TAKING YOUR HEALTH IN YOUR HANDS

If somebody had given you a fine car or a fine house, you'd want to maintain it. If the car weren't firing right, you'd want to get somebody under the hood to fix it. If your house needed paint, you'd paint it. You wouldn't want these things to go to wrack and ruin because they are valuable.

When it comes to the body, we sometimes seem more careless of the gift. Often that means paying no attention to the body until it acts up. Sometimes, by then, it's too late. Sometimes, even though we can still get it fixed, the repairs are costly, they take time, they may bring our lives to a temporary halt.

That's why the first step is yours to take. Essentially, it means maintenance. If you're a smoker, what you're doing is roughly what you might do to your car if you put sugar in the tank. You are causing malfunctions. If you're addicted to drugs or drinking too much, you are causing malfunctions. If you have a lot of sexual partners, you're risking serious breakdowns. Even if you sleep with one stranger and don't use a condom, you're acting as you might if you took that car down a busy highway at 90 miles an hour.

Diet is another part of maintenance that you can take care of. Too many of us eat poorly, live on junk food, get fat, and don't eat enough fiber to rid our bodies of poisons that can accumulate. Not thinking about what you put into your body is recklessness. It means you don't care. Not thinking about what you put into your family's bodies is even worse recklessness. It shows you don't seriously care about the people you love.

Diets aren't as complicated as the steady barrage of new diet books might make you think. The basic principles are simple: eat low-fat foods and lots of fresh fruits and vegetables, raw as well as cooked. The fruits and vegetables help clear your body of something called free radicals, which can damage the cells' genetic material and cause trouble in your circulatory system. Fats clog your blood vessels and can increase the likelihood that you'll get cancer—as well as diabetes and other diseases. Your body needs some fat, of course. But there are better sources for it than greasy meat and butter. Substitute fish for meat whenever you can. Omega-3 fatty acids in fish oils, also found in soybeans and certain nuts and seeds, are good for you. They lower your cholesterol instead of raising it. Use canola or olive oil for cooking. Both are excellent in helping you lower blood cholesterol.

Diet is one part of a larger picture. One meaning of health equality must be your right to know as much about health and disease as the next person, even if the next person happens to be white. Sometimes it is hard to disentangle race from economics. Somebody remarked that America is the only country where the poor are fat and the rich are lean. The truth behind this is that people with more money and more education are likely to know more about taking care of themselves.

But you don't *have* to be rich to get this knowledge. Check out the Web site of Hilton Publishing (*www.hiltonpub.com*) for health tips as well as delicious low-fat soul food recipes. If you don't have a computer, go to the library. Your local librarian can help you find the site and show you how to print out the recipes.

We talked about diet as a key to disease prevention. Exercise is another urgent part of body maintenance. Lots of us are active— maybe even hyperactive—when we're kids, but then we slip into becoming couch potatoes. The results? Look at it this way. To go back to that fine auto you inherited, leave it in the garage for a few months and you'll find you have lots of new troubles. Maybe the battery's dead. The tires are mushy. The fuel line is clogged with gunk.

The body is like a car: it's meant to be used. Your heart needs to work. So do your lungs. Adult or child, you have to work to get rid of fat that otherwise will build up and cause troubles. If you're taking in a lot of fats and not exercising, you're risking disease.

Exercise is easy. Take a brisk walk every day for half an hour or so. Go to a gym if you can. Play ball in your local playground. You'll be surprised to find that not only will the pounds slip away but so will the years. Nothing is better for stimulating the body than good exercise. It's also the best path to a vigorous old age. We know people in their seventies and even their eighties who, because they exercise regularly, still move around as if they were twenty years younger, and enjoy their lives with great gusto. Exercise is good for your body, to be sure. But it's also good for your soul: once it becomes a habit, it will make you feel good.

LEARNING A LITTLE MEDICINE

A larger aspect of health maintenance is knowing your body—how it works, how it doesn't work, and how to put it right if it goes wrong. If we had our way, everyone in this country would get a basic medical education in the public schools. All the reading and writing and arithmetic in the world won't do you much good if you're sick all the time and can't make use of your knowledge.

You've started that education already by reading this book. There are many excellent books out there. We recommend as a good place to start a book by Neil Shulman, M.D. that you can find in the drugstore or your local bookstore: it's called *Your Body's Red Light Warning Signals* (New York: Dell Publishing, a division of Random House, Inc., 1999), and it gives you medical tips that can save your life. *The Black Man's Guide to Good Health* (Hilton Publishing, 2001: Roscoe, IL), which has plenty of good information for women, too, is another excellent source. It gives you the basic knowledge you need about prevention, disease, and treatment.

Know your body— how it works, how it doesn't work, and how to put it right if it goes wrong.

Learning how your body works and how it doesn't work when it's diseased is obviously good in itself. It will help you stay healthy. It will help you know when you are seriously ill and what to do about it. It will also help you communicate with doctors, which, as you know, can be most important.

When you talk to your doctor, you will want to present your symptoms as clearly as you can. At the same time, you will want to understand clearly what the doctor has to say about your diagnosis and treatment. It may help if you take with you a list of the things you want to find out from the doctor, such as:

- What your doctor thinks your problem is
- Whether you should take further tests in order to arrive at a firm diagnosis
- Once that diagnosis is certain, what the treatment options are—including the advantages and disadvantages of each
- What the prognosis is, and if favorable, how long you must continue treatment before you start to get well
- How likely cancer is to return even after effective treatment
- What the cost of your treatment will be beyond what your insurance covers, if you have insurance. If you have none, you want to know if there are local, state, or federal agencies that can help you pay for your treatment. Often, in such cases, your primary-care provider will be Medicaid. Medicaid works just like an HMO, but it works for people without insurance or other means to pay medical bills. If you're on Medicaid, read through the pamphlets and know how it works.

You'll naturally have other questions of your own to ask. *Write them down.* That way, when you're in the office with your physician, you won't get rattled and forget to ask what you need to know.

There are still other things you can do to prepare for your visit to the doctor and to help it go as well as possible:

- Keep a detailed record of how you're feeling, so you can clearly report to the doctor any changes that are happening in your body.
- Bring a friend or relative with you. Visits to a doctor can be emotionally trying, especially if you're sick. Having a friend with you can help you better remember what the doctor tells you.
- If you don't understand something the doctor tells you, ask questions.

- If the doctor suggests a treatment plan, ask if there are alternatives.
- If you don't come away satisfied that you clearly understand the options, see a second doctor. The more radical the treatment, the more important it is that you know clearly its advantages and disadvantages, and the alternatives, if there are any.

We wish we could solve the disparities in medical treatment between blacks and whites by just writing about them. Obviously, we can't. Neither can we make sure that you have your own doctor. Not everyone has the money for that. Finally, we can't guarantee that when you do get to see a doctor, that doctor will suit you. But we hope and expect that he or she will treat you with the dignity and attention you deserve.

What we can do is insist that to some extent it's within your own power to stay healthy or, should you fall ill, to get timely and proper treatment to put you on the road to recovery. In the end, it's your body. You must accept responsibility for keeping it finely tuned.

TWENTY-TWO

Surgery and the Body-Mind Connection

CANCER OFTEN MEANS SURGERY, and surgery always means pain. Though a surgeon's cut is made as an act of healing, I am the first to admit it is also a deep and painful wound. I say this with intimate knowledge because I have experience both as the person holding the knife and as the one under the knife.

Five times I have lain on my back under the bright lights of the operating room. Five times I've felt myself go under anesthesia on that narrow table, and five times I've awakened to pain. Even when, formally speaking, my surgeries were "minor," as they were in two instances, they felt major to me.

For the patient, *no* surgery is minor. Even a biopsy, given under local anesthetic, can feel serious, as one lies, awake, waiting for the instrument to cut away a bit of one's flesh, however small that bit may be.

SURGERY AND THE SPIRIT

Those are the hard facts. But thankfully, we don't live only in a world of facts. We have spirit, too, and in my experience it is the spirit that gets us through our difficult times. For me, the spirit's strength is the belief in God. That means, on the patient's part, a willingness to hand over one's life not just to the surgeon's art but to the power of God's love as well. For me as a surgical patient this has meant the same spiritual action I take each time I grasp a scalpel—I pray that God may guide my thoughts and actions, and the outcomes as well.

For the patient, no surgery is minor.

The form that prayer has taken for me in the operating room, as it does in my daily life, is "Lord, I am in your hands. Thy will be done." There are moments in our lives when no other stance is adequate or appropriate. The feeling that comes when we hand over our lives in that way is something like what a child feels in its mother's comforting arms.

Most of us know the fuller version of that prayer in which we hand our being over to the keeping of God. I refer to Psalm 23, which for me has been a comforting prayer against cancer:

"The Lord is my shepherd. I shall not want. He makes me to lie down in green pastures; He leads me beside the still waters. He restores my soul; He leads me in the paths of righteousness for His namesake. Yea, though I walk through the valley of the shadow of death, I will fear no evil; for You are with me. Your rod and Your staff, they comfort me. You prepare a table before me, in the presence of my enemies; You anoint my head with oil; my cup runs over. Surely goodness and mercy shall follow me all the days of my life, and I will dwell in the house of the Lord forever."

My wife's favorite biblical passage is Psalm 51 which begins:

"Have mercy upon me, O God, according to your loving kindness; according unto the multitude of your tender mercies, blot out my transgressions."

This prayer has carried her, as my prayer has carried me, through more than one ordeal.

ADDITIONAL PRAYERS

- Our God, our Father, we ask a special prayer this morning. Enter _____'s body today and give him/her the strength to withstand the surgery and provide him/her with thine healing powers. Be with Dr._____ and his team of physicians. Guide their hands and direct their decisions. If it is your will, have it so that our loved one will return safely to this room. These blessings we ask through Jesus Christ, our Lord. Amen.

- Once again, dear Lord, we turn to you for strength, for understanding and patience. Once again, be with Dr. _____ and his surgical team. Be with _____. Give him/her the courage to return to surgery. Amen.

PRAYERS FOR THE CANCER PATIENT

- Heavenly Father, in the quietude of my soul, dissuade my fears of helplessness, hopelessness, and despair. Instill within me the serenity that you gave Daniel in the lion's den and David as he faced Goliath. As I face that dreaded disease, cancer, descend upon me with all your healing power, I pray thee. If it be your will, exorcise from me the cancer which exists within me. Return me to your vineyard to do your earthly work. Amen.

- Everlasting and almighty God, I know that all power of healing rests with thee. If it is your will, remove this cancer from my body, I beseech thee. Amen.

- Everpresent and omnipotent God, we honor and glorify thee. We observe the simple ant and the powerful elephant. We note the howling winds, the warm sun and needed rains. Rid this cancer from my body, I beseech thee. Guide my treatment. Renew my spirit and make me whole to do your work here on earth. Amen.

Some of these prayers my wife offered for me when I entered surgery to have my thyroid removed.

SUGGESTED SCRIPTURES

The Scripture	The Need
Psalm 46	To face a crisis
Isaiah 40	When discouraged
Psalm 91	Facing illness
Psalm 107	Family and friends in difficulty
2 Timothy 3	Major difficulties
Hebrews	Trust in God
1 Corinthians 15	Bereavement
Revelations 21	Bereavement
Psalm 27:14	When facing difficulty
Psalm 34:19	When suffering an affliction
Psalm 49:15; 23:4	Certainty of death
Luke 23:46	Certainty of death
Ephesians 6	Equipment for difficulties
Joshua 1:9	Help in all cases

For all the times you may have heard and said these prayers and scriptures, they are never more real than in that moment when you say them silently before you are put to sleep in the surgery room. Saying Psalm 23 has prepared me to endure what I had to endure. I have awakened to pain and known what it's like to dread coughing or swallowing because they mean more pain. I know what it's like to be unable to urinate or defecate. But I know also that to stand close to a force greater than myself brought me a comfort stronger than the pain and discomfort.

UNDERSTANDING YOUR
MEDICAL SITUATION

In regard to surgery as to so much else, the Lord helps those who help themselves. I mean that long before you get to the operating table, you have a job to do that requires your intelligence, patience, and courage.

In an earlier chapter, we talked about how maintaining your body meant paying it the same attention you'd bring to maintaining a car. But, of course, a patient isn't a commodity, like a car brought to the garage to be fixed. For the car, we must assume, having one's radiator replaced is not a soul-wrenching experience. But you are a conscious agent, so it's important for you to prepare for surgery by learning in advance as much as you can about why it's necessary and what you must expect. Once you've learned this, you can accept the surgery because you have *chosen* to do it. That means that you will not bring to the operating table that extra stress of fear or even panic, and that your body will be better able to withstand and recover from the ordeal.

Prepare for surgery by learning in advance as much as you can and why it's necessary and what to expect.

Learning starts with questions. Since you've read this far, you know what those questions are, but let's look at them again, if only as review:

- Are there other options and, if so, what are they, what do they promise, and what do they risk?
- Is the surgery "curative"? Some operations are designed for less than that—to give the patient more physical comfort, for example, or to get a better look at the extent of the cancer.
- What are the risks; are potential complications reversible, and are they life threatening?
- How long will it be before you can get back to your ordinary life, and even when you do, what changes—like giving up

smoking, eating a healthier diet, or exercising more—will be required of you?

You'll have many more questions, I'm sure. The essential thing to know is that, though in the past surgeons may have been reluctant to discuss such matters with patients, today surgeons know that you, as a living, thinking person, want to understand your case as clearly as a layperson can.

Communication with your surgeon requires that he or she explain the medical procedures in clear, simple language.

Communication with your surgeon requires that he or she explain the medical situation and the procedures in clear, simple language. If your surgeon doesn't do that, simply say that you don't understand, and ask for a clearer explanation. If the surgeon is then unwilling or unable to explain more clearly, you may wish to seek a second opinion—an opinion that would include the clear explanation you need.

Many people decide to seek a second opinion as a matter of course. You know already that the decision to operate or not is based on a number of complicated diagnostic observations, on the stage of

Speaking to a second specialist may help you come to a decision with which you're comfortable.

the cancer, and on the patient's general health. There are times when the advantages and disadvantages of surgery may balance very closely. Speaking to a second specialist may help you come to a decision with which you're comfortable. Even if, as is most often the case, it is the same decision you made in the first place, your affirmation will be stronger, and you will have greater confidence in the decision when you know that two specialists have independently arrived at the same conclusion.

It's good also if you can consult a surgeon or surgeons whom others—your minister or family or friends—have strongly recommended. You have every right to learn as much as you can about the person who is going to perform surgery on you. You have the right to know how many such surgeries he or she has performed, how many of these were successful, and how many have not been. Of course, you will want to ask such questions politely. Insist, however, on answers.

Learning as much as you can about your condition and its treatment, becoming confident (sometimes through second opinions) that the therapy you have chosen is the best for you, and having confidence in your surgeon—these are the steps that will ease your mind as far as it can be in difficult circumstances.

Surgery is a realm where the medical and spiritual worlds come together. If you bring worry into the operating room, it means greater stress for you. We don't want to suggest that very many patients go through surgery without any anxiety. But if, at that moment before the anesthesia sets in, you're unsure in your heart whether you're doing the right thing, your stress level is likely to be especially high. That means that your blood pressure will go up and your immune system will be weaker.

Soothing your spirit before surgery is not simply good religion—it is also good medicine.

Soothing your spirit before surgery is not simply good religion—it is also good medicine. Your job is to know as much as you can, to bow your spirit to the necessity you decided on, and to have faith that God will guide the surgeon in his thoughts and technical maneuvers.

THE SPIRIT'S MANY FORMS

Because I am a Christian, I have put special emphasis on that spiritual form. But the spirit knows many forms, and I certainly don't think one must be a Christian in order to get through surgery successfully. In David Bognar's *Cancer: Increasing Your Odds for Survival* (Salt Lake City: Hunter House, 1998), I read a fascinating interview with Joan Borysenko, Ph.D., a cell biologist who, when her own father died of leukemia, decided that she did not "want to work with isolated cells anymore." That was when Dr. Borysenko entered Harvard Medical School to study behavioral medicine with Dr. Herbert Benson.

Behavioral medicine means, essentially, that the mind and body are intimately connected. What happens to each will affect the other. Stress is a mental–emotional–spiritual problem that, if we bring unresolved to the operating table, can cause serious trouble for us. This means that the patient preparing for surgery will want to calm the mind as far as possible.

Dr. Borysenko observes that when the mind relaxes—that is, becomes relatively free of stress—several favorable changes occur in the body. The heart rate goes down, and so does blood pressure. Certain hormonal changes occur as well, and so do changes in brain wave patterns.

Researchers like Dr. Borysenko have made large claims for the benefits of such relaxation techniques:

- The techniques strengthen the immune system.
- They help the body to fight cancer and even slow the growth of tumors after they've developed.
- They reduce anxiety and depression.
- They reduce the discomfort and pain that can follow from surgery.

I'm an old-school doctor, trained to be skeptical of such claims. Skepticism, after all, is the way science works to sharpen our thinking about things. But I also know through my experience with Christian prayer that when I can put my fears to rest, I suffer less. So I want to outline some of the relaxation methods that have worked for others and may work for you.

MEDITATION

Meditation is a simple technique. It requires only half an hour a day of your time. People of every faith have attested to its benefits for thousands of years. These days, in major cities, meditation centers are easy to find, and many of them offer free or inexpensive instruction. But the basic principles of meditation are simple enough, and you can at least begin to practice them without instruction.

Pick a time of day and a place that are reasonably quiet and free from telephone calls and other distractions. Sit on a thick cushion on the floor, legs crossed, or in a straight-backed chair, keeping an upright posture so your back is not supported by the back of the chair. Your spine, neck, top of your head, should all be in a line, as though someone were pulling you up with a string attached to the top of your head. In other words, sit tall.

Sit still, resting your hands palms down on your thighs. Rest your eyes also, using a soft gaze, on a point about five feet ahead of you on the floor. Keep it there but gently, without fixing your focus. Locate your breathing in your abdomen. You can do this by pushing your breath all the way out on the exhale and then sending your awareness to the intake and outtake of your breath. Do this for ten or so breaths until you've located your breathing. Then just breathe naturally, without trying to breathe in any special way, but being aware of your breathing as it goes in an out of its own accord.

You might begin meditating by sitting for ten minutes a day, or ten minutes twice a day, and then lengthen the time as you get used to the practice. Set a timer so you don't need to watch the clock. You will notice as you sit that your mind produces an endless stream of images, worries, plans, meals, daydreams, and so on, both positive and negative. They race in one after another. No doubt your anticipation of the surgery will be an important part of that parade of images.

At the beginning stage, the realization of your mind's energy that spins out thoughts randomly can be shocking and disagreeable. This is what the Buddhist's call "monkey mind" or "grasshopper mind," for obvious reasons. But meditation trains the mind to regard this endless stream as a passing show, no one thought more important than another. When you find yourself getting caught up in your plans for the day or fantasies, or worries about surgery, just label this "thinking" and return your awareness to your breathing, to the present moment, to where you are sitting in a room.

The point is to stay alert yet also relaxed, letting thoughts come and go. Meditation is sometimes falsely looked at as a way to "clear your mind." You will not clear it but learn to regard it in a different way.

It is more important to maintain a continuity of practice from day to day than to sit for longer periods of time. For example, sit for ten minutes every day when you get up, rather than for thirty minutes on Monday and then not again until Thursday.

IMAGERY

One of the writers of this book has a friend who has lived for eight years with an ovarian cancer that, even after she'd been treated by surgery and chemotherapy, her physicians believed would kill her within a year. Our friend, who is a fighter, wasn't willing to spend that year waiting to see what happened. She'd heard of cases where a macrobiotic diet helped others control their cancer, and she decided that if it worked for others, she'd make it work for her. She went on the diet and has been on it since, and she's still alive—not cancer free, but vital and happy and hopeful. So we recommend that you take a closer look at that diet as we outlined it in Chapter 3.

Even while our friend was keeping her diet, she practiced a technique that involves imagery. When the cancer had metastasized to her lungs, she imagined the cancer as vividly as she could. And she imagined it growing smaller. She practiced this imaging technique daily for half an hour each day, beginning with a relaxing technique, then imaging. The cancer that had appeared on her lung in fact vanished. Today, though she isn't free of cancer, she continues to manage it with courage and focus and good-heartedness.

She remembers that a few days before the x-ray confirmed that the cancer on her lung *had* vanished, she imagined her white corpuscles in a kind of congo line, carrying out on a tray held over their heads the last of the defeated cancer cells. I wish you could see her describe this, the twinkle in her eye, and the little shake of her body that she gave when the congo line got to the sixth beat. May God give us all something of her spirit.

AFFIRMATIONS

Today, affirmation is a widely used technique in psychotherapy. You'll find it described in David Bognar's *Cancer: Increasing Your Odds for Survival.* Affirmation involves replacing a harmful, established, negative belief about the self with a healing positive one. We have many case histories suggesting that people with negative self-images can be given new confidence by this method.

Some cancer patients have been helped by therapists familiar with this technique. We don't pretend that it's easy to fashion affirmations around cancer or around the surgery we might need in order to cure it. It is possible, however. The method will work best under the guidance of someone who can make us face our fears even as we reach down for our strengths.

MUSIC THERAPY

A number of major hospitals today offer music therapy as a complementary therapy. Music therapy can be used in connection with imagery guided by a therapist to relieve anxieties and fears. Some patients have found that it helps them lessen the nausea and vomiting that normally accompany chemotherapy.

If you're interested in this relaxing technique, you may wish to call the American Music Therapy Association at (301) 589-3300 for information and referrals.

HUMOR

Some years back, the writer Norman Cousins wrote a book called *Anatomy of an Illness as Perceived by the Patient* (Bantam, 1981) in which he recounted a remarkable story. Cousins had been diagnosed with a progressive spinal disease, and he'd been told he had only 1 chance in 500 to recover. Hearing that, Cousins checked out of the hospital and into a hotel, where he treated himself with Marx Brothers movies and some old Candid Camera shows. Watching the shows and deliberately seeking out other ways to make himself laugh was for Cousins a deliberate experiment. He believed that laughter and positive thoughts were medicines in themselves.

For Cousins, it worked out that way. Laughter gave him relief from pain and made sleep possible. Whether or not laughter also *cured* Cousins, perhaps no one can say. But he did recover from the disease.

Cousin's story was so compelling that he went on to teach the technique at the UCLA medical school, and to lecture widely about body–mind medicine.

TWENTY-THREE

If You Must Have Surgery

I'VE ALREADY TOLD YOU something about the moment I became a different kind of surgeon—a wounded healer, if you will. It happened on the morning when I first detected a lump in my neck. I knew at once what it was. I'd felt a hundred such lumps in my own patients. Now, a little to my astonishment, this tumor was in me.

My mind then went from the tumor to the percentages—15 to 25 percent of these tumors are malignant. Could be a lot worse. But to tell you the truth, though I'd offered such numbers to patients many times in the hope that the numbers would ease their minds, they didn't ease mine much.

I went to work that morning, after arranging to have my tumor examined. That evening, I was scheduled to play bridge in a tournament, and I decided to go ahead with that, too. Maybe I was just trying to delay as long as I could a hard moment I knew lay before me. I didn't play well that evening. More than once my hand went to the lump, hoping to find it had gone away.

My wife was asleep by the time I got home. Obviously, I didn't have to tell her that night. Telling the family about my illness was a hard thing. I'd been a strong man all my life. That's how my family saw me, a man of steel. Now the healer who so many times had tried to lift the spirits of his patients, needed lifting himself. I was a mortal man with a tumor.

The next morning I couldn't put it off any longer. My wife was shocked, but not for long. She arranged for me to tell the news to our daughters.

I'd always known that surgery was a family affair. Only family and loved ones can bring the right smile, the right touch, the right tear, the right word, to the patient in need of loving concern from others. Sometimes I've had patients who had to go through surgery alone, and it struck me then what a hard thing that was—to be alone in a time of such need.

Make your case a family affair.

So I made my case a family affair. I opened myself to my wife's and my daughters' love and concern, and I felt stronger for having done it. I encourage you to do the same.

SELECTING A MEDICAL TEAM AND CHOOSING BETWEEN TREATMENT OPTIONS

Before the first day of my awareness was over, I had set the second step in motion also. For me this was relatively easy. I simply called a surgeon I knew and trusted. But for most patients, selecting a medical team in whom one has confidence is a big job. Often, the process begins with the family doctor's recommending the specialists he or she believes in. Another way to begin is to follow leads provided by friends or relatives who may have been treated by surgeons and other cancer specialists in a humane and skillful fashion.

If you don't have a family doctor and don't have other leads to follow, call your local hospital and tell them what you need. They'll tell you how and where to get started.

SECOND OPINIONS

An increasing number of hospitals provide what are called *multidisciplinary second opinions*. This means that instead of your recommended treatment coming from one doctor, it will come from a panel of specialists. To find such a hospital near you, call the National Cancer Institute: 1-800-4-CANCER. They can also give you information on a specific type of cancer.

If you don't have the benefit of multidisciplinary second opinions, a single second opinion is still an option that offers several excellent advantages:

- It gives you a chance to learn more about your disease and its prognosis. When you talked to the first specialist, you were probably frightened and unable to take in everything you were told.
- It often gives you a clearer understanding of the treatment options.
- It gives you time to know in your heart that you've made the right choice.

David Bognar, in *Cancer: Increasing Your Odds for Survival,* reports that in one major cancer center, 70 percent of patients who sought a second opinion made changes in their treatment as a result of that consultation. Sometimes this meant that the patient found a doctor more congenial; sometimes a more attractive option was recommended by the second doctor.

In the first wave of fear that usually follows a diagnosis of cancer, you may feel panicky and rushed, and wish to start treatment as quickly as possible. But the vast majority of these cases are *not* driven by such emergency. Of course, you must not delay too long. But you definitely *can* take time to think it through—which means getting hold of as much information as you can.

In brief, here are the tasks you face after being diagnosed with cancer:

- Open yourself emotionally to family and friends.
- With the help of your family doctor and what you can learn from friends who have gone through cancer treatment, select a medical team and decide on treatment.
- Learn to manage stress.
- Invite God's love through prayer.

DEALING WITH FEAR AND PAIN

So there they are—the two hard things that fall on the cancer patient right at the start—(1) to share the news with family and loved ones, and to do so in such a way that news of illness strengthens the ties rather than weakens them; and (2) to educate yourself to your medical situation through reading, conversations with specialists, and discussions with friends who have been through what you must go through. This education will also include the second opinion.

But as you know already, there are still further emotional and practical ordeals that cancer patient must go through—fear of the operation and of the pain that goes with it, the ordeals of postoperative therapy and recovery, and the fear of death itself. Add to this the disruptions brought about by cancer treatment, the time missed from work, even the possibility of losing one's job.

Even when the operation and recovery phase are over, there remains the five-year waiting period. I'm sorry to say that even then the cancer can return. I know this all too well. My own did, seventeen years after the successful operation on my thyroid!

Some people come through these ordeals with flying colors. I'm sure you know some of them. They're stronger than they were before they got cancer. Not only do they take better care of themselves—getting exercise and paying attention to what they eat—but they have a depth of character that comes only to those who have been through the fire.

In my own experience, it has been the men and women who have an appetite for life, a flame in the soul that flares up to the wonder of each day, in sickness and in health, who come through these ordeals most strongly. Remember that a hunger for life doesn't have to rest on a fear of death. Sometimes in America you feel that's the best guarded secret that we have—that we die. I'm going to talk about this more directly in the next chapter, but let me say now that all of us need to come to terms with our mortality. That's a humbling experience, to be sure, and for many of us it's a frightening one. But I'm convinced that it's those who have somehow wrestled with it and found a way to make an odd gentleman's (or gentle lady's) agreement with it who are best able to hold their heads up in adversity. And sometimes, as I'd find for myself when I feared I might lose everything I loved, coming into that agreement gives us a passion for the moment that is the salt of life. You'll remember the text: "This is the day that the Lord has made. Let us rejoice and be glad in it." (Psalm 118:24, King James Version)

CHRISTIAN FAITH AND CANCER

I must say a few words more about the way my own Christian faith has helped me cope with cancer. It's what I believe, and it's what has worked for me. If you aren't a Christian, you may still find for yourself some version of the spiritual process I describe here. It's as close as I can come to speaking about the psychological, emotional, and spiritual transformations that add up to the kind of courage I admire in others.

My own minister at the Whitherspoon Presbyterian Church in Indianapolis preached recently on the adage "Let go. Let God." A certain kind of people do best living with cancer. They are best able to come back after surgery, get through chemo and x-ray therapies with the least damage, and return to their normal lives. And they seem to draw their strength from something beyond the ego.

To be sure, these survivors are often strong-willed people. They do everything they can to help themselves, before and after treatment. (Often, interestingly, they have also done much to help oth-

Learn to live day by day; you'll often find the days feel richer.

ers.) But in addition they are able to come to terms with their destiny, by admitting that the outcome of their illness lies outside their power to determine. They learn to live day by day, and often they find that the days feel richer that way.

I know that some Christians think of their cancers as an expression of God's wrath against their sin. It's been just the opposite for me. In my suffering, I've found that God willingly sent his grace to demonstrate his love.

He has done this for me whenever I was able honestly and openly to surrender myself to him through prayer, sacrifice, and love. Once I had learned to give myself up to him in this way, I felt a heavy load lifted from my shoulders. When that load of grief and fear melted away, I felt joy. I was glad to be alive. I was grateful to be in God's hands.

For me, seeking God's love, communing with him, means prayer. In prayer, I empty my heart, my soul, and my thoughts of apprehension. In prayer, my fearful thoughts are supplanted by his serenity. Only when, as sometimes happens, I stray from the path of daily prayer does that human frailty of guilt disguised as anxiety and hopelessness return.

One keeps hope alive in the face of cancer through the unbounded resourcefulness of the human spirit. We have great powers to call on. To illustrate these more widely, I'll tell you a story.

Back in the summer of 1995, my wife, Lu, and I were attending a Vacation Bible School. My daughter, Bette-Jo, had come out to drop her daughter off, but when she saw me she ran back to her car, weeping. In my absence, she'd received the MRI report on her mother in the office where she practices as an eye doctor. And now she had to face me with it.

My wife had been complaining of increasing back pain. It had gotten bad enough to require a mild narcotic. So we'd decided to get to the bottom of it. The diagnosis my daughter had received reported "extensive metastatic cancer of the lumbar spine." Bette Jo and I exchanged glances: we both knew what

One keeps hope alive in the face of cancer through the unbounded resourcefulness of the human spirit.

that meant. It meant that Lu probably had no more than six months to live. There was a good chance that her spine would collapse and leave her paralyzed. She might require around-the-clock nursing. Bette-Jo and I didn't talk about those fears—not then. Each of us knew what the other was thinking, and we were thinking the same thoughts.

Instead, we walked back to the fellowship hall, where Lu was telling a story. She's a born storyteller, with a clear and loving voice, an artist's eye for the right detail, and an actor's ear for the right emphasis.

As we entered the hall, she'd already started telling the story of the paralytic man whose friends brought him to Christ to be healed. That odd coincidence made me listen to her especially intently. You know the story. When some of the people around Jesus wouldn't let the paralyzed man in, his friends lowered him through an opening in the roof to lay at Jesus' feet. "Your sins are forgiven," Jesus said, and the man was healed.

As I listened to Lu, I was thinking back over our life together since we met at Florida A&M University. Over the years, I'd had the chance to appreciate more and more her love of life and her talent for living it, her sincerity and unselfishness, and that happiness that she seemed to carry with her whatever she did, wherever she went, whomever she was with. Had I been taking those remarkable gifts too much for granted?

For years, Lu had been after me to go to the movies with her, but I'd rarely had time. She wanted to go fishing with me, too, but I'd always found fishing boring, so I'd say I was too busy, or that the day wasn't right, or that I didn't know where to get worms. That moment in the prayer hall I remembered the lake my barber had told me about, stocked thick with trout. We'd go there—next week, once we'd taken care of medical matters. I thought of the movies now playing, and how I'd give her a menu, let her say which one we'd see.

Years ago, I'd begun a speech with a quotation from an unknown source:

"Do not keep the alabaster box of your love and tenderness sealed up until your friends are dead. Speak approving, cheering words while their ears can hear them and while their hearts can be thrilled and made happier by them. Postmortem kindness does not cheer the burdened spirit. Flowers on the coffin cast no fragrance backward over the weary way."

We were all ready to find ways to express our love. Lu had given hers so unstintingly. As my younger daughter had told her more than once, "Mom, you're what makes this family click."

Lu's story has a happy ending. I was skeptical about the diagnosis. Lu hadn't lost weight; she wasn't anemic. She'd had a mammogram, chest x-ray, and colonoscopy within the past three months, and they'd all come out fine. True, there could be cancer in areas that these tests hadn't revealed, but I knew I must talk to the radiologist.

It turned out that he *had* made a mistake—never mind exactly how. Technicians are human; so are the systems of information they operate in. So on occasion technicians and that system may fail.

This time, the results of that failure turned out to be a happy one. Lu took a round of tests that didn't come up with a specific diagnosis but made a malignancy look very unlikely. Somehow, both

Lu and I came away from that experience drawing the same conclusion. We began to do at least some of the things we probably should have been doing earlier. We made our lives together still more rich, by taking time to do things we both enjoyed—travel, shopping, golf. We went to a few movies. We even intend to go fishing as soon as our arthritic limbs permit.

The lesson we drew from all this was easy, and we think it's a good lesson, with or without cancer: live the days and weeks and months and years as if they were your last. We've found that this stance brings out the best in us—the best of love, the best of hope, the best enjoyment of life, as it unfolds moment by moment.

KEEPING HOPE ALIVE WHEN CANCER RECURS

In particular cases, doctors can't know why cancer returns, but we do have general ideas. Maybe the original treatment was incomplete—the surgery didn't catch everything, or the therapy that followed was ineffective. Maybe the immune system wasn't strong enough to suppress the cancer.

You know already that cancer's a subtle beast. A cell is somehow modified genetically, and an aspect of its changed condition is that it can change other, healthy cells to become like it. Out of that uncontrollable multiplication of cells comes a kind of change in the body. The modified cells, which at a certain point form a mass we call a tumor, no longer operate according to the rules that keep the body's system balanced and harmonious. If cancer is allowed to grow without medical intervention, it has the power to sabotage the body's fundamental life systems.

The fact is that for some people the fight against cancer may go on over a long lifetime. They will have long periods when they feel good and appear healthy by the measure of all available medical tests. But somehow, hidden, the cancer has remained dormant in them, presumably held in check by a strong immune system. Should that immune system be weakened, however—say, by sickness or stress—the sleeping enemy awakens and resumes its cruel work.

All this brings me to another story.

TONY JONES'S STORY

I'd known Tony Jones for years. He'd more than once called me about medical problems, real or imagined. He'd always bring up the medical question only after we'd talked for a while about other things, as a kind of afterthought.

This time Tony talked about his business for a while. I was always a ready listener, curious about a life so different from mine. Then he switched gears. He'd had a pain in his right side for several days and was afraid it might be appendicitis.

When we brought him in for tests, it looked as if he might be right. His temperature was elevated, he had a high white count (over 12,000), and the pain was on the right side. The presumptive diagnosis—the one we make before we have *all* the information—was appendicitis, and that meant surgery.

Tony didn't like the idea of the operation, but I was able to persuade him that we had no choice. His condition was already potentially dangerous. Once we went in, we found that his appendix was indeed inflamed, but that was a secondary problem. The real trouble was a nearby tumor.

When a surgeon goes in looking for one thing and finds another, he needs to discuss the matter with the patient and loved ones. They've given permission for one kind of procedure. They must decide whether to permit another, often more extensive, one. What made the surgery I recommended for Tony more drastic is that it meant I'd have to remove a segment of his colon. Because we couldn't biopsy the tumor *before* removing it, it was always possible that the tumor I removed might prove benign. But benign or not, the tumor was already making Tony sick, and it had to be removed.

Tony's wife accepted my view of the situation. We talked about whether Tony himself should decide, but under the circumstance, that made no sense. It would mean that we'd have to wait until Tony had recovered from anesthesia. It would also mean sewing him up and then cutting again.

The procedure went smoothly. What we found was that besides the cancer of the cecum (right colon) with obstructive appendicitis that I'd already come across, the cancer had also entered neighboring lymph nodes.

Tony came out of the operation very well. After completing chemotherapy, he returned to his old life, and he felt and appeared perfectly healthy. Then, during a regular checkup, Tony learned that his x-ray showed a round shadow in both lungs. Again I operated. This time, entering through incisions on both sides of the chest, I removed the target areas. As we thought, the pathologist reported that Tony's biopsy sample disclosed the type of cancer that had originated in the colon.

This meant that, though for a second time we removed the visible cancer, neither Tony nor I could be sure that it wouldn't strike later, in some unpredictable place.

I'd always thought of Tony as a bit of a worrier. He'd lived a busy life and had never taken much time to look around. But the first bout of cancer taught him something. He'd found a better balance between his family and his work. He even started trying things he'd never have tried before, like joining a reading group at the public library.

In any case, something had changed in him. I was pleased to see that a couple of months after the operation he seemed cheery. He wasn't asking of me any guarantees I couldn't give him. He seemed to accept the situation as it was.

That was ten years ago. Tony has experienced no further battles with cancer. He's retired now, at a sufficiently ripe age, and he likes to play, sometimes on the golf course, sometimes with his grandson. Once a week he goes down to the high school to meet with a boy he's mentoring. He and the boy have become great pals.

CARE GROUPS

I've been talking about support the patient must draw from his or her individual soul. I've said something also about support loved ones can draw from one another. But I haven't talked yet about the support we get through the company of others who are in the same boat.

John Riley was in a dreadful state when he learned that prostate surgery had left him impotent. Then his doctor steered him to a care group. The group helped John come to terms with his loss. They also shared resources they'd found that sometimes helped their sexual enjoyment and performance. Following his friends' lead, Jake even did some reading. What he said to me when I last saw him was this: "I'll tell you, Doc, there are things we weren't meant to do alone. Sometimes I think all that John Wayne, Wesley Snipes stuff makes us a little crazy."

Care groups can be infinitely resourceful. Mable Berry, after she'd had a breast removed, joined a group called Reach. Twice each month they meet to show off their new exercises, to keep each other *doing* their exercises, to compare their various experiences with implants and other prosthetic devices, and to call for and give each other emotional support.

Mable hasn't found it easy, even with all that help, to decide which way to go about prosthesis. Her friend Sally, whom she met in the group, shows her own surgically created breast, for Mable's admiration. "Yes, Sally," Mable says, "they've certainly done a fine job with you. But for me it's still the question whether I want another trip under the knife. I guess I'll just stick to my "Susy.""

Nothing pleases me more than to see cancer patients who once were blind but now can see. When it comes to exercise, they find any number of ways to do it. For some, it's a routine they perform each morning when they wake up. Some people enjoy going to a YMCA or health spa. But lots of the people I know in these groups like to do things together—walk in a park or a mall, bowl, play golf. When John Riley heard people in his group complain that there wasn't a decent place in the neighborhood to take a walk, he organized a walk in the local mall each Monday, Wednesday, and Friday, four miles each day.

These groups are also excellent at sharing diet news between the members. Mable got so interested in the subject of diet that she had her friend Dot Harper, a dietician, give the group a kind of mini-course in diet. They learned the importance of a diet low in fat and high in fiber. They talked about how to cut down meat and increase the use of fish. From Dot, they learned something about the differences between HDL and LDL, and between saturated and unsaturated fats. Before the course was over they knew something about vitamins, what you get from a healthy diet, and what you might wish to get in supplements. Believe it or not, several of them could talk pretty knowledgeably about oxidants and antioxidants, too.

What I find exciting about these "new dieticians," if I can call them that, is that they help not just their own health but the health of their families, too. When the cooking changes in the family, people may howl a little. But in the long run, the new dieticians' knowledge and conviction will prevail. After all, it's easy enough to make tasty and filling food that isn't full of poisons.

As it happens, both John Riley's group and Mable's invited a member of the American Cancer Society to speak on the importance of not smoking. Sorry to say, some of the members were still having trouble stopping. What the speaker told them was enough to convince them. Once you know what smoking and chewing tobacco do to your body you'll stop— unless they're stupid or suicidal.

Care groups can become quite intimate, to the point where members can share their deepest fears about death and pain and loss. So that's what our book must look at next.

CONCLUSION

For many people, especially those who catch it early, cancer is like other diseases: it is diagnosed, it is treated, and it is cured. But for others, it is something that comes and goes, and sometimes comes again. Even among this second group, there are people who get cured, or who at least live comfortably for a long time. But there are also those, and we know there are many, who will die of it. These we can only keep as comfortable as possible for as long as possible.

We think that the individual's temperament has a bearing on whether or not he or she finds a way to live with cancer. Some people are defeated by it emotionally, and when that happens, they are more likely to be defeated physically as well. Our families, our friends, our care groups, our own souls, and our faith are all important resources for those who must live with cancer.

TWENTY-FOUR

Living with Cancer

YOU KNOW ALREADY the importance of a strong spirit for the patient who is managing cancer. Now we must turn to the more difficult question of how to sustain the spirit even in the shadow of death.

Certainly, one of the first thoughts that flash before the minds of patients just diagnosed is "Am I going to die?" In many cases, of course, the answer is no; in others, it is yes. People die, and some people die of cancer.

Dying of cancer is a special kind of death. It is not sudden as is a massive heart attack, a stroke, or an auto crash. Where death attends such cases, there's little or no chance to say good-bye. Even more important, there's no chance to put one's soul in order.

If anything good *can* be said about cancer, it's that it sometimes feeds the spirit by testing it. People find courage and other resources during their ordeal. They learn to look with a peculiarly open eye at the loss of everything they love. Yes, people can grow in the very act of dying even though they may also shrink into sorrow and anger.

DENIAL OF DEATH

One of the hard things about preparing for death is that most of us invest a lifetime in denying that death can touch us. Lately, I looked over a very good book on physical and emotional well-being addressed to black women. I found marvelous discussions of self-esteem and acting effectively. I found very helpful chapters on reproductive issues, and on the diseases most likely to strike black women. But I didn't find so much as an index reference to death.

Most of us invest a lifetime in denying that death can touch us.

Death needn't be a closely guarded secret, but in our culture it often appears to be. Most people don't want to talk about it or think about it, let alone read about it. We fear death as a mystery not even science is likely to bring into the open. We dread the idea that we may cease to be. We dread the unspeakable loss—the loss of everything, a loved one's smile, a child at play, all the memories and sheer existence that belong to each one of us, and will now perhaps vanish from the universe.

Science would say that as individuals we vanish, but our molecular particles live forever. Christians and others say that the soul lives on in an afterworld of paradise for the good and hell for the bad. Buddhists say that the self is subject to incarnation, either upward or downward on the ladder of consciousness, and that it is in this way immortal.

Even among those who believe that some part of our individual awareness goes on after death, there are a thousand schools of thought on just what that "going on" might be.

The one thing about death that the majority of human beings do agree on is that one's own death sentence is abrupt and unfair. Sure, other people die. But us?

Death *is* unfair. Sometimes we must die when we do not have time to die, whether this means we're too young or we're old but still enjoying things. Death is unfair. Sometimes people stay frightened all the way through dying; for them it will never be the right time.

People have always been frightened of death and, sometimes, out of their fears, we have made great tribal stories. Many scholars, for example, see the fall from Eden as a tale that explains death. Early people couldn't think of death as a natural thing any more than we can. They were sure that it must be a form of divine punishment. Even today, I've had patients who consider it that way. Though it isn't the way I take it.

Doctors aren't strangers to death, but for us too it's a hard subject. Doctors sometimes think of death as a failure. We fight for the lives of our patients as long and hard as we can. If they die, we review what we did, hoping we don't find a mistaken or an omitted action that helped cause the death.

Although doctors are likely to view death from a purely scientific perspective, even to scientists, death remains something of a mystery. A particular enzyme ceases to function or some amino acid is rearranged in DNA to lead the body's tissues and systems down the pathway to death.

But to speak of death is to speak of a medical process that is also a divine secret. I think that it's good it is a mystery, and I pray it will remain so. Should that mystery ever be unwrapped by science, you may be sure that there will follow a strong campaign to eliminate death. In my mind, such a step would mean more of a disaster to us than even nuclear war. In both cases, we will have seized powerful forces far too strong for our management. This is why I rejoice that for the while, at least, death remains a divine mystery. I rejoice too that for me the heart of that mystery is eternal life.

PAIN AND PAIN MANAGEMENT

One reason we fear death is that we fear pain—both the anticipation and the actuality. Dying of cancer can mean great pain. Often a patient will have gone through surgery and other therapies that themselves cause pain and discomfort. Perhaps an organ or body system has been invaded by inoperable cancer. That can mean great pain, which, left unattended, will increase as the terminal cancer runs its course.

One reason we fear death is that we fear pain.

Yet pain, through pain management, can be controlled. For the terminal cancer patient, pain management requires that we make the patient as comfortable as possible while he or she passes through the death process.

Doctors begin pain relief, or management, using mild pain relievers. If these fail to control the pain, stronger ones are used. At some stages, at least, and for some people, drugs like Extra-Strength Tylenol® or Advil® may be strong enough. If the pain becomes more intense, a mild narcotic like codeine with Tylenol might suffice. But as the disease becomes more intensive and aggressive, the patient will need strong pain-killers like demerol or morphine. At each stage the patient and loved ones will wish to weigh physical comfort against the fact that, with deepening sedation, the patient will be more completely lost to himself or herself and to the loved ones.

Through pain management, pain can be controlled.

Many people prefer to remain clear and conscious for as long as possible. For each person, the point when increased sedation is needed will be different. Most doctors feel that a patient should not be left in acute suffering if medicine can help. Sometimes patients add to their suffering out of fear of becoming addicted. True, occasionally, even in cases that appear to be terminal, people *do* recover, addicted. But freeing oneself of addiction is a relatively minor problem in this context.

MEDICAL INTERVENTION

How far medicine can intrude in cases of terminal cancer only the patient and loved ones can decide. We hope they will decide on the basis of a clear understanding of the medical situation.

At a point when sustaining life can *only* mean additional suffering, you may, with your loved one's medical team, decide to have all life-support systems, even nutrition, stop. Sometimes the patient will have stipulated this in his or her living will.

Death is a process. For each of us, there comes a moment when we must simply allow it to happen.

HOME CARE VERSUS HOSPITAL CARE

Where death occurs is often a matter of choice. Some people prefer to die at home. For this to be possible, there must be a strong and organized support system. It is nearly impossible for one person to do the job alone. Dying continues through a twenty-four-hour schedule. Getting through that schedule can exhaust a team, even when they have outside support. The dying patient will require nursing and bathing; linen has to be changed often; pain medication has to be administered and monitored. Equally important, family members must stay close to the patient, talk with them, and let them know that they are loved.

Where death occurs is often a matter of choice.

If you choose to care for your loved one at home, the hospital or your local libraries can help you find a service called *hospice,* or you may get information directly by calling (800) 854-3402 or (202) 638-5419 or sending an e-mail. Hospice will provide you with assistance from trained people—some of them nurses—who specialize in helping others die with reasonable comfort and dignity. Incidentally, once the patient is *terminal*—that is, has given up traditional medical treatment (chemo, radiation, and hospital treatment) and means of lengthening life, Medicare covers nearly all hospice expenses.

Hospice workers help you to rearrange a room to accommodate a hospital bed, if that's necessary. They'll show you how to change linen while the dying person is in the bed. They'll help you with administering medicine, and show you how to assist the patient to evacuate waste when necessary. They are especially skilled at pain management. But, maybe most important, they will bring to the experience of dying a dignified, yet at the same time light-hearted, spirit. The purpose here is not to fight death but instead to surrender to it.

Family members must stay close to the patient and let them know they are loved.

Hospice is not for everyone. The patient may prefer the hospital, even feel more secure there. In the hospital, the patient can assume that everyone knows what he or she is doing. Home care, even with hospice assistance, may not always inspire that confidence.

But it is also true that home care means that the patient can be surrounded by family love in a home environment. The patient can enjoy social life in its final phase—the saying of good-byes, which can often mean not only tears but also smiles and laughter. The patient can be surrounded by what gives him or her spiritual comfort.

Hospice care means that the patient and loved ones are ready to acknowledge the inevitability of this death. Traditional medical care means staying in the hospital, medical intervention when necessary to keep the patient alive, and the use of drugs to control disease, even when they cannot cure it. As hospice spokespeople themselves put it, such an approach is the right one as long as cure is possible. It may even be the right one when cure *isn't* possible. But it is not the only choice.

Hospice care is a choice you make to enhance life for a dying person. With the support of hospice, a person with a terminal disease may choose to die at home with the loving help of family, friends, and caring professionals. Hospice care emphasizes comfort measures and counseling to provide social, spiritual, and physical support to the dying patient and his or her family. All hospice care is under professional medical supervision.

WAITING FOR DEATH

We all know the question: what would you do if you had only six months to live? Or three months, or two? Some people make this a gracious time. They continue doing what they always did for as long as they can support it. They find a way to live through each stage of their decline with a quality of acceptance and peace.

We can only think of this as a high spiritual accomplishment, this strength to go through the ultimate ordeal without losing the human attributes of sweetness and grace.

PREPARING FOR DEATH

While the patient is still alert, and the earlier the better, there are decisions to make:

- Whether to die in the hospital or at home
- Whether to allow medical treatment that will keep the patient alive past the point where there is any chance for recovery or for conscious life
- How to dispose of property
- Whether to donate organs
- Who will care for the surviving family?
- Who will pay the bills?
- Who will take over my business?

- What form should the funeral ceremony take?

And so on.

All these questions are complicated and none can be taken lightly, but by dealing with them the dying person has the opportunity to take control of his or her own death. These questions can be resolved long before you fall ill, through *wills, living wills,* and *health care proxies.* These documents tell people specifically what you want to happen after your death: who gets what parts of your property or wealth, how long you want medical support, whether you wish to donate any of your organs, and much more.

If you haven't faced them already, you will have to face some of these questions during a terminal illness. Of course, you also have the option of *not* addressing them, and thus leaving your dying in the hands of others. If you make that choice, though, you should understand that your wishes may not be carried out the way you'd like. These are difficult human choices, and no one, except the person making them, is in a position to say what is the right course for him or her.

Some people may wish to avoid the ordeal of long drawn-out sickness when the only possible outcome is death. They may request in a living will not to allow medical intervention beyond a certain point. Patients have the right to refuse medical treatment in any situation. By thinking through such questions in advance, you make it more likely you will be able to make the best decision for yourself.

You can also make your wishes known in the form of an *advance medical directive.* If your health care institution will not honor your wishes, federal law obliges them to tell you so upon admission. But the fact is that doctors and nurses almost always do just what the family and the patient want.

Yes, dying can be complicated. It can mean finding answers to hard questions. But for many black people, and I for one, at the heart of the matter is a common faith. Many of us have heard the powerful words from the mouth of a dying loved one: "I'm going to be with my God." That is a faith that can give the dying person courage and make him or her whole.

TWO VOICES OF EXPERIENCE

I am more aware of a mystery and beauty in life since I have accepted death as a personal eventuality before me. Before then, I had thought of death out there; now I know that I am going to die. That has released me for more vivid living. I reach out more. Almost everything reminds me of its connections with other things. My present is many-textured. I do not look to the future with dread. It has to be shorter than my past but it does not have to be less rich.

—A 78-year-old woman[*]

A thought has come to me in the last few years. I doubt that when I die my life will be over—my life with all its loving and caring and striving. Can it be that all my loved ones—mother, sister, other relatives—can all this love be gone? Nothing in nature disappears. Out of our bones, our skeletons, new life comes in some other way.

—An 85-year-old woman[*]

That death can bring a new richness is a hard thought to accept, but many people, men as well as women, have experienced this. What it requires of us is courage and forethought. Resources are available to help you find both.

---

[*] These two stories are reprinted with permission from the Boston Women's Health Book Collective, *Our Bodies, Ourselves for the New Century,* New York: Touchstone/Simon and Shuster, p. 580.

EPILOGUE

We wrote this book out of our faith that knowledge is power. We wrote it to tell you how to live in a way most likely to prevent cancer from invading your body. We wrote it also to tell you, should you be stricken by cancer, how to recognize its signs, how to get the best medical help, and even how to rearrange your life as a recovering cancer patient in ways that will best feed your courage and resolution and faith.

There are health disparities in America that make it harder for African Americans and others to get the kind of medical care that every American deserves. Till those disparities end, however, you aren't helpless. You've learned a great deal about what you can do to help yourself.

We think that a cure for cancer can be found. Some very promising drugs are being tested, and other routes are being explored as well. But till the time comes when there is a cure for cancer, African Americans, like other Americans, must become soldiers in the fight against it. Let us enter the fight armed with knowledge.

RESOURCES

CHAPTER 1

National Cancer Institute, "What You Need to Know About Cancer"
www.nlm.nih.gov/medlineplus/ency/article/001289.htm
NIH, Medline Plus Medical Encyclopedia
www.nlm.nih.gov/medlineplus/print/ency/article/000374.htm

CHAPTER 2

American Cancer Society. *Cancer Facts and Figures 1996*. Atlanta, GA: American Cancer Society, 1996.

Dollinger, Malin, et al. *Everyone's Guide to Cancer Therapy*. Kansas City, MO: Andrews McMeel Pub., 1998.

Williams, Wendy. *The Power Within: True Stories of Exceptional Patients Who Fought Back with Hope*. New York: Simon & Schuster, 1991.

CHAPTER 5

Books

Boston Women's Health Collective. *Our Bodies, Our Selves for the New Century.* New York: Simon & Schuster, 1998.

Kelly, Patricia T. *Understanding Breast Cancer Risk.* Philadelphia: Temple University Press, 1991.

Lord, Audre. *The Cancer Journals.* San Francisco: Aunt Lute Books, 1997.

Organizations

American Cancer Society
Toll-free: (800) 227-2345
Web site: www.cancer.org/docroot/home/index.asp

National Cancer Institute
9000 Rockville Pike
Building 31, Room 4A-18
Bethesda, MD 20892
Toll-free: (800) 4-CANCER
Web site: www.cancer.gov

Cancer Research Institute
681 5th Avenue, 12th Floor
New York, NY, 10022
Toll-free: (800) 9-CANCER
Web site: www.cancerresearch.org

American Institute for Cancer Research
1759 R Street NW
Washington, DC 20009
Toll-free: (800) 843-8114
Web site: www.aicr.org

CHAPTER 6

The National Institute of Health Web site:
www.meds.com/pdq/colon_pat.html
CancerNet (a service of the National Cancer Institute) Web site:
cancernet.nci.nih.gov/Cancer_Types/Colon_And_
Rectal_Cancer.shtml

Colon Cancer Alliance
1440 Coral Ridge Drive
Suite 386
Coral Springs, FL 33071
Telephone: 877–422–2030
Fax: (425) 940–6147
Web site: www.ccalliance.org/what/contact/contact.html

CHAPTER 7

Lung Cancer Online Home Page, www.lungcanceronline.org/
(guides you to physicians, hospitals, HMOs, lung cancer
programs, second opinions, etc.)
National Cancer Institute: Lung Cancer
Web site: www.cancer.gov/cancertopics/types/lung

CHAPTER 9

National Cancer Institute, "Thyroid Cancer" Web site:
www.cancer.gov/cancertopics/types/thyroid

The National Cancer Institute
9000 Rockville Pike
Building 31, Room 4A-18
Bethesda, MD 20892

Telephone: (800) 4-CANCER; (301) 435-3848
Web site: www.cancer.gov

American Cancer Society
1599 Clifton Road, N.E.
Atlanta, GA 30329
Telephone: (800) ACS-2345
Web site: www.cancer.org/docroot/home/index.asp

CHAPTER 10

National Cancer Institute: Endometrial Cancer Web site:
    www.cancer.gov/cancertopics/types/endometrial

CHAPTER 11

National Cancer Institute: *What You Need to Know About Cancer of
    the Cervix.* Available from the National Cancer Institute, Office
    of Cancer Communications, 31 Center Drive, MSC 2580,
    Bethesda, MD 20892; (800) 4-CANCER
Posner, Tina, and Martin Vessey. *Prevention of Cervical Cancer.*
    London: Kings Fund Publishing Office, 1988. Available
    through the Kings Fund Centre, 126 Albert Street, London
    NWI 7NF, U.K.

CHAPTER 12

American Cancer Society. "Ovarian Cancer." CA 45, no. 2 (1995):
    Special issue.
Piver, M. Steven, and Gene Wilder. *Gilda's Disease: Sharing Personal
    Experiences and a Medical Perspective on Ovarian Cancer.*
    Amherst, NY: Prometheus Books, 1996.

CHAPTER 19

You may find a full list of resources in *Our Bodies, Ourselves* (New York: Touchstone, 1998). Here is a brief sample:

Probably the best way to start is to call (800) 458-5231, the toll-free National AIDS Clearing House, a branch of the CDC. They will refer you to the AIDS organization nearest you.

There is a national AIDS hotline you can reach by calling (800) 432-AIDS (Spanish: (800) 344-7342; TTY (800) 243-7889.) Open every day, 24 hours a day, the hotline will provide you with information and refer you to a local organization.

For prison resources, contact AIDS Counseling and Education (ACE), Bedford Hills Correctional Facility, 247 Harris Road, Bedford Hills, NY 10570; (914) 241-3100, ext. 260. You may also contact the National Prison Project, 1875 Connecticut Avenue NW, Suite 410; Washington, DC 20009; (202) 331-0500.

CHAPTER 21

AMA, Ethics and Health Disparities. Available at www.ama-assn.org/ama/pub/category/9421.html

CHAPTER 22

Patch Adams. *Gesundheit! Bringing Good Health to You, the Medical System, and Society through Physician Services, Complementary Therapies, Humor, and Joy.* Rochester, VT: Inner Traditions International, 1998.

David Bognar. *Cancer: Increasing Your Odds for Survival.* Salt Lake City, UT: Hunter House, 1998.

Mind/Body Health Sciences, Inc.
393 Dixon Road
Boulder, CO 80302
Telephone: (303) 440-8460
Offers programs on use of mind to benefit the body.

Kushi Institute of the Berkshires
Box 7
Becket, MA 01223
Telephone: (413) 623-5742
Offers programs on macrobiotic diet and lifestyle changes.

CHAPTER 23

National Cancer Institute: Toll-free: (800) 4-CANCER

CHAPTER 24

Choice in Dying
200 Varick Street
New York, NY 10014-4810
Telephone: (212) 366-5540
This group advocates recognizing and preserving individual rights
at the end of life.

Hospice Foundation of America
2001 S Street NW, Suite 300
Washington, DC 20009
Phone: (800) 854-3402 or (202) 638-5419
Fax: (202) 638-5312
E-mail: info@hospicefoundation.org
Web site: www.hospicefoundation.org

SELECTED BIBLIOGRAPHY

Chapter 1

Cecil, Russell L. *Textbook of Medicine,* 20th ed. Philadelphia, PA: W. B. Saunders Co., 1991, pp. 32–36.

Clayton, L. L. A., and W. Byrd. "The African American Cancer Crisis. Part I: The Problem," *Journal of Health Care,* 1993, 4:83–101.

Cooley, M. et al. "Lung Cancer in African Americans: A Call for Action," *Cancer Practice,* 1998, 6–12.

Denniston, R. "Cancer Knowledge, Attitudes and Practices Among Black Americans." *Progress in Clinical and Biological Research,* 1981, 53:225–235.

Freeman, H. P. "Affirmative Action in the Diagnosis and Treatment of Cancer in Blacks." American Cancer Society Science Seminar.

Hamilton, Edwin. *The Health and Wellness Ministry in the African American Church,* Longwood, FL: Xulon Press, 1994.

Leffall, L. D. "Program Priorities for the Future: Cancer Among Black Populations," *Progress in Clinical and Biological Research,* 1981, 53:253–263.

Myers, M. H. et al. "Contrasts in Survival of Black and White Cancer Patients, 1960-73." *Journal of the National Cancer Institute,* 60:1209–1215.

Parker, S. L. et al. "Cancer Statistics, 1997." *CA: A Cancer Journal for Clinicians,* 1997, 47:5–27.

Powe, B. D. "Cancer Fatalism Among Afro Americans: A Review of Literature." *Nursing Outlook,* 1996, 44:1821.

Underwood, S. M. "Cancer Risk Reduction and Easily Detected Behaviors Among Black Men: Focus on Learned Helplessness." *Community Health Nursing,* 1992, 9:21–31.

Chapter 2

Benett, J. C., and F. Plum, eds. *Cecil Textbook of Medicine,* 20th ed., Philadelphia: W. B. Saunders, 1996.

Schwartz, Seymour I. et al., eds. *Principles of Surgery,* 6th ed., New York, NY: McGraw-Hill, Inc., 1994.

Chapter 3

American Institute for Cancer Research. "Diet and Cancer Report. Food Nutrition and the Prevention of Cancer: A Global Perspective," pp. 1–8. Available at: <www.aicr.org/>.

American Institute for Cancer Research. "Food, Nutrition and the Prevention of Cancer," Available at: <www.aicr.org/>.

Arnot, B., *The Breast Cancer Prevention Diet,* Revised & Updated, Boston: Little, Brown and Co., 1999.

Balch, C. M. et al. "Oncology." In: Schwartz, S. I. et al., eds. *Principles of Surgery,* 6th ed., New York: McGraw-Hill, 1994, pp. 305–76.

Bland, K. I., and E. M. Copeland III. "Breast." In: Schwartz, S. I. et al., eds. *Principles of Surgery,* 6th ed., New York: McGraw-Hill, 1994, pp. 531–593.

Bland, K. I. et al. "Analysis of Breast Cancer Screening in Women Younger Than Fifty Years of Age." *Journal of the American Medical Association,* 1981, 245:1037.

Bland, K. et al. "National Cancer Data Base," *Cancer Annual: Review for Cancer Patient Care,* 1998, pp. A35–A46.

Bland, K. I. et al. "In-Situ Carcinoma of the Breast: Ductal and Lobular Cell Origin." In: Cameron, J. L., ed. *Current Surgical Therapy,* 4th ed., St. Louis, MO: Mosby Year Book, 1992, pp. 612–621.

Browman, G. "Evidence-Based Paradigms and Opinions in Clinical

Management and Cancer Research." *Seminars in Oncology,* 1999, 26(8):9–13.

Cady, B., et al. "Evaluation of Common Breast Problems: Guidance for Primary Care Providers." *CA, A Cancer Journal for Clinicians,*1998, 48(1):49–60.

Crajdos, C. et al. "Lymphatic Invasion, Tumor Size, and Age Are Independent Predictors of Axillary Lymph Node Metastases in Women with T1 Breast Cancer." *Annals of Surgery,* 1999, 230(5):692–696.

Cummings, S. et al. "The Effect of Raloxefene on Risk of BRCA in Postmenopausal Women." *Journal of the American Medical Association,* 1999, 281(23):2189–2197.

Early Breast Cancer Trialists Collaborative Group. "Systemic Treatment of Early Breast Cancer by Hormonal Cytotoxic or Immune Therapy. 133 Randomized Trials Involving 31,000 Recurrences and 24,000 Deaths Among 75,000 Women." *Lancet,* 1992, 339:1.

Fernandez, E., et al. "Fish Consumption and Cancer Risk." *American Journal of Clinical Nutrition,* 1999, 70(1):85–90.

Fisher, B. "Lumpectomy (Segmental Mastectomy) and Axillary Dissection. In Bland K. I., and E. M. Copeland III, eds. *The Breast: Comprehensive Management of Benign and Malignant Diseases.* Philadelphia: W. B. Saunders, 1991, pp. 634–652.

Fisher, B. et al. "Ten-Year Results of a Randomized Clinical Trial Comparing Radical Mastectomy and Total Mastectomy with or with- out Radiation." *New England Journal of Medicine,* 1974, 312(11):674.

Fremgen, A. M. et al., "Clinical highlights from the National Cancer Data Base 1999." *CA, A Cancer Journal for Clinicians,* 1999; 49:145-158.

Gapstur, S. et al. "Hormone Replacement Therapy and Risk of Breast Cancer with a Favorable Histology." *Journal of the American Medical Association,* 1999, 281(22):2091–2047.

Hamilton, E. H. *The Health and Wellness Ministry in the African American Church,* Longwood, FL: Xulon Press, 1994.

Hartman, L. C. et al. "Efficacy of Bilateral Prophylactic Mastectomy in Women with a Family History of Breast Cancer." *New England Journal of Medicine,* 1999, 540(2):77–84.

Jeffrey, S. et al. "Radiofrequency Ablation of Breast Cancer. First Report of an Emerging Technology." *Archives of Surgery,* 1999, 13:1064–1068.

King, Dean et al., eds. *Cancer Combat.* New York, NY: Bantam Books, 1998.

Kinnon, J. "New Breast Cancer Threat." *Ebony,* October 1999, pp. 52–59.

Kurer, H. et al. "Incidence and Impact of Documented Eradication of Breast Cancer Axillary Lymph Node Metastases Before Surgery in Patients Treated with Neoadjuvant Chemotherapy." *Annals of Surgery,* 1999, 22(1):72–78.

Lewis, B., and R. McConry. "Breast Cancer." In: Benett, J. C., and F. Plum, eds. *Cecil Textbook of Medicine,* 20th ed., Philadelphia: W. B. Saunders, 1996, pp. 1320–1325.

Lundgren, S. "Prospects in Endocrine Treatment of Breast Cancer." *CA, A Cancer Journal for Clinicians,* [n.d.], 7(6).

Morton, D. L. et al. "Clinical Review of the Sentinel Node Hypothesis." *Surgery,* 1999, 126(5):815–819.

Nasholtz, J-M. "The Role of Toxins in the Managements of Breast Cancer." *Seminars in Oncology,* 1999, 26(8):1–3.

Rawlings, P. A. et al. "Factors Correlated with Progression-Free Survival After High-Dose Chemotherapy and Hematopoietic Stem Cell Transplantation for Metastatic Breast Cancer." *Journal of the American Medical Association,* 1999, 282(14):1335–1343.

Roses, D. et al. "Complications of Level I and II Axillary Disease in Treatment of Cancer of the Breast." *Annals of Surgery,* 1999, 230(2):194–195.

Secundy, Marian Gray et al. *Trials, Tribulations, and Celebrations: African-American Perspectives on Health, Illness, Aging and Loss.* Yarmouth, ME: Intercultural Press, 1992.

Seldman, A. "Single-Agent Paclitaxel in the Treatment of Breast Cancer: Phase I and II Development." *Seminars in Oncology,* 1999, 26(3):14–20.

Serdula, M. K. et al. "Prevalence of Attempting Weight Loss and Strategies for Controlling Weight." *Journal of American Medical Association,* 1999, 282(14):1353–1358.

Shulman, Neil, M.D., James Reed, M. D., and Charlene Shucker. *The Black Man's Guide to Good Health.* Roscoe, IL: Hilton Publishing, 2001.

Staren, E. et al. "Ultrasound-Guided Needle Biopsy of the Breast." *Surgery,* 1999, 126:629–635.

Veronesi, U. et al. "Radiation After Breast Preserving Surgery in Women with Localized Cancer of the Breast." *New England Journal of Medicine*, 1993, 328:1587.

Winchester, D. P., and J. Cox. "Standards for Diagnosis and Management of Invasive Breast Cancer." *CA, A Cancer Journal for Clinicians*, 1998, 1:108–109.

Winchester, D. P., P. Strom, and C. A. Eric. "Standards for Diagnosis and Management of Ductal Carcinoma In-Situ (DCIS) of the Breast," *CA, A Cancer Journal for Clinicians*, 1998, 48(2):108–128.

Wong, J. et al. "Lymphatic Drainage of Skin to a Sentinel Lymph Node in Feline Model." *Annals of Surgery*, 1991, 214:637–641.

Chapter 4

Arnot, Dr. Bob. *The Breast Cancer Prevention Diet*. Boston: Little, Brown and Co., 1999.

Kushi, Michio. *The Macrobiotic Approach to Cancer*. Garden City Park, NY: Avery Publishing, 1991.

Chapter 6

Levin, Bernard, "Neoplasms of the Large and Small Intestine." In: Benett, J. C., and F. Plum, eds. *Cecil Textbook of Medicine*, 20th ed., Philadelphia: W. B. Saunders, 1996, pp. 713-721.

Chapter 7

Benowitz, N. "Tobacco." In: Benett, J. C., and F. Plum, eds. *Cecil Textbook of Medicine*, 20th ed., Philadelphia: W. B. Saunders, 1996, pp. 33–36.

Blot, W. "The Epidemiology of Cancer." In: Benett, J. C., and F. Plum, eds. *Cecil Textbook of Medicine*, 20th ed., Philadelphia: W. B. Saunders, 1996, pp. 1013–1017.

Bridge, P. "A Strategy for Monitoring Program Integrity in a Statewide Tobacco Prevention Health Education Program." *Journal of Cancer Education*, 1999, 14(3):73.

King, T., and Smith, C. "Chest Wall Pleura, Lung and Mediastinum." In: Schwartz, S. I. et al., eds. *Principles of Surgery*, 6th ed., New York: McGraw-Hill, 1994, pp. 737–749.

Miller, Y. "Pulmonary Neoplasms." In: Benett, J. C., and F. Plum, eds. *Cecil Textbook of Medicine*, 20th ed., Philadelphia: W. B. Saunders, 1996, pp. 436–442.

Omenn, G. "Cancer Prevention." In: Benett, J. C., and F. Plum, eds., *Cecil Textbook of Medicine*, 20th ed., Philadelphia: W. B. Saunders, 1996, pp. 155–156.

Schneider, C. P. "Eighth World Conference on Lung Cancer, August 10–15, 1997, Dublin, Ireland," *Journal of Cancer Research*, 1998, 124:62–64.

Chapter 8

Harlan, L. et al. "Geographic, Age, and Racial Variation in the Treatment of Local/Regional Carcinoma of the Prostate." *Journal of Clinical Oncology*, 1995, 13:93–100.

Mettlin, C. et al. "The National Cancer Data Base Report on Prostate Carcinoma After the Peak in Incidence Rates in the U.S." *Cancer Annual: Review of Cancer Patient Care*, 1998, AS47–AS52.

National Cancer Institute. *Prostate Cancer*, NIH Publication No. 96-1576. Revised June 1996.

Peters, P. C. et al. "Urology: Prostate Cancer." In: Schwartz, S. I. et al., eds. *Principles of Surgery*, 6th ed., New York: McGraw-Hill, 1994, pp. 1762–1765.

Pettaway, C. A. "Racial Differences in the Androgen/Androgen Receptor Pathway in Prostate Cancer." *Journal of the National Medical Association*, 1999, 91:653–660.

Chapter 9

Chin, B. et al. *Management of Solitary Thyroid Nodules*. Display at American College of Surgeons, San Francisco, October 1999.

Dillman,W. "The Thyroid," In: Benett, J. C., and F. Plum, eds. *Cecil Textbook of Medicine*, 20th ed., Philadelphia: W. B. Saunders, 1996.

Hundahl, S. et al. "A National Cancer Data Base Report on 53,856 Cases of Thyroid Carcinoma Treated in the U.S., 1985-86." *Cancer*, 1998, 83:2638–2648.

Kaplan, E. "Thyroid and Parathyroid Principles of Surgery." In: Schwartz, S. I. et al., eds. *Principles of Surgery*, 6th ed., New York: McGraw-Hill, 1994, pp. 1611–1680.

Mozzeferri, E.L. Personal communication.

National Cancer Institute. *Cancer Facts: Questions About Thyroid Cancer*, 1998. Available at: <www.cancer.gov/>.

Chapter 10

American Cancer Society. *Cancer Facts and Figures* 2000. Available at: <www.cancer.org/docroot/STT/content/STT_1x_2000_Facts_ and_Figures.asp>.

Chen, F. et al. "Differences in Stage at Presentation of Breast and Gynecological Cancers Among Whites, Blacks, and Hispanics." *Cancer,* 1994, 73:2838–2842.

Connell, P. et al. "Race and Clinical Outcome in Endometrial Carcinoma." *Obstetrics and Gynecology,* 1999, 94(5):713–720.

Hicks, M. L. et al. "The National Cancer Data Base Report on Endometrial Carcinoma in African-American Women." *Cancer,* 1998, 83(12):2629–2637.

Howell, E. et al. "Differences in Cervical Mortality Among Black and White Women." *Obstetrics and Gynecology,* 1999, 94(4):509–515.

Kohler, M. P. et al. "P53 Overexpession in Advanced-Stage Endometrial Cancer." *American Journal of Obstetrics and Gynecology,* 1996, 175:1246–1252.

Otten, M.W., Jr., et al. "The Effect of Known Risk Factors on the Excess Mortality of Black Adults in the United States." *Journal of the American Medical Association,* 1990, 163:845–880.

Rogers, R., and G. Sutton. "Endometrial Cancer." In: Schwartz, S. I. et al., eds. *Principles of Surgery,* 6th ed. New York: McGraw-Hill, 1994, pp. 1813–1815.

Chapter 11

Chen, F. et al. "Differences in Stage at Presentation of Breast and Gynecological Cancers Among Whites, Blacks and Hispanics." *Cancer,* 1994, 73:2838–2842.

Cusick, J. "Human Papillomavirus Testing for Primary Cancer Screening." *Journal of the American Medical Association,* 2000, 83:109–109.

Howell, E. et al. "Differences in Cervical Mortality Among Black and White Women." *Obstetrics and Gynecology,* 1999, 95:A04:509–515.

Niazi, M. "HIV and Cancers" (poster). American College of Surgeons, October 1999, Bronx Lebanon Hospital Center, Bronx, NY.

Rogers, R., and G. Sutton. "Carcinoma of the Cervix." In: Schwartz, S. I.

et al., eds. *Principles of Surgery,* 6th ed. New York: McGraw-Hill, 1994, pp.1809–1813.

Wright, T. C. et al. "HPV DNA Testing of Self-Collected Vaginal Samples Compared with Cytologic Screening to Detect Cervical Cancer," *Journal of the American Medical Association,* 2000, 283:81–93.

Wright, T. C. et al. "Human Papillomavirus Is a Necessary Cause of Invasive Cervical Cancer Worldwide." *Journal of Pathology,* 1999, 189:12–19.

Chapter 12

Peters, P. et al. "Neoplasms Renal Parechymal Tumors." In: Schwartz, S. I. et al., eds. *Principles of Surgery,* 6th ed., New York: McGraw-Hill, 1994, pp. 1757–1764.

Chapter 13

Peters, P. et al. "Urology: Urinary Bladder." In: Schwartz, S. I. et al., eds. *Principles of Surgery,* 6th ed., New York: McGraw-Hill, 1994, pp. 1761–1764.

Shapiro, C. et al. "Tumor of the Kidney, Ureter and Bladder." In: Benett, J. C., and F. Plum, eds. *Cecil Textbook of Medicine,* 20th ed., Philadelphia: W. B. Saunders, 1996, pp. 623–626.

Chapter 14

Peters, P. et al. "Neoplasms Renal Parenchymal Tumors." In: Schwartz, S. I. et al., eds. *Principles of Surgery,* 6th ed., New York: McGraw-Hill, 1994, pp. 1757–1764.

Chapter 15

Peters, J., et al. "Esophagus and Diaphragmatic Hernia." In: Schwartz, S. I. et al., eds. *Principles of Surgery,* 6th ed., New York: McGraw-Hill, 1994, pp. 1043–1122.

Chapter 16

Moody, Frank et al. "Stomach." In: Schwartz, S. I. et al., eds. *Principles of Surgery,* 6th ed., New York: McGraw-Hill, 1994, pp. 1123–1152.

Chapter 17

National Institute of Health. "Cancer of the Pancreas," NCI Publication No. 96-1560, April 1996.

Reber, H. "Tumors of the Pancreas." In: Schwartz, S. I. et al., eds. *Principles of Surgery,* 6th ed., New York: McGraw-Hill, 1994, pp. 1421–1429.

Chapter 19

Centers for Disease Control and Prevention. "Critical Need to Pay Attention to HIV Prevention for African Americans," HIV/AIDS Fact Sheet, 1998.

Coleman, J. J. III, and M. Sultan. "Tumors of the Head and Neck." In: Schwartz, S. I. et al., eds. *Principles of Surgery,* 6th ed., New York: McGraw-Hill, 1994, p. 649.

Curan, J. "Epidemiology of HIV Infection and AIDS." In: Benett, J. C., and F. Plum, eds. *Cecil Textbook of Medicine,* 20th ed., Philadelphia: W. B. Saunders, 1996, pp. 1846–1851.

Scadden, D. T., and J. E. Croiopman. "Hematology/Oncology in AIDS." In: Benett, J. C., and F. Plum, eds. *Cecil Textbook of Medicine,* 20th ed., Philadelphia: W. B. Saunders, 1996, pp.1870–1875.

Soag, M. "Prevention of HIV Infection." In: Benett, J. C., and F. Plum, eds. *Cecil Textbook of Medicine,* 20th ed., Philadelphia: W. B. Saunders, 1996, pp. 1851–1855.

Chapter 20

Applebaum, F. "The Acute Leukemias." In: Benett, J. C., and F. Plum, eds. *Cecil Textbook of Medicine,* 20th ed., Philadelphia: W. B. Saunders, 1996, pp. 936–940.

Hook, E. "Chancroid Syphilis." In: Benett, J. C., and F. Plum, eds. *Cecil Textbook of Medicine,* 20th ed. Philadelphia: W. B. Saunders, 1996, pp. 1704–1714.

Keating, M. "The Chronic Leukemias." In: Benett, J. C., and F. Plum, eds. *Cecil Textbook of Medicine,* 20th ed., pp. 925–935.

Peters, P. et al. "Carcinoma of the Penis." In: Schwartz, S. I. et al., eds. *Principles of Surgery,* 6th ed., New York: McGraw-Hill, 1994, p. 1765.

Peters, P. et al. "Testicular Tumor." In: Schwartz, S. I. et al., eds. *Principles of Surgery,* 6th ed., New York: McGraw-Hill, 1994, pp.1764–1765.

Portlock, C., and J. Yahlom. "Hodgkin's Disease." In: Benett, J. C., and F.
    Plum, eds. *Cecil Textbook of Medicine,* 20th ed., New York: McGraw-
    Hill, 1994, pp. 947–954.

Chapter 21

Abraham, L. K. *Mamma Might Be Better Off Dead: The Failure of Health
    Care in Urban America.* Chicago: U. of Chicago Press, reprint edition,
    1994.
Council on Ethical and Judicial Affairs. "Black-White Disparities in
    Health Care," *Journal of the American Medical Association,* 1990,
    263:2344–2346.
Dula, A., and S. Goering. *It Just Ain't Fair: The Ethics of Health Care for
    African Americans.* Westport, CT: Praeger Publishers, 1994.
Louis Harris & Associates. "National comparative survey of minority
    health care." The Commonwealth Fund. 1995. Available at:
    <www.cmwf.org/publist>.
Minority Affairs Consortium. American Medical Association."Racial and
    Ethnic Disparities in Health Care," Reports of the Board of Trustees,
    AMA Reference Committee on Amendments to Constitution and
    Bylaws. 2003. Available at: www.ama-assn.org/ama/pub/cate-
    gory/6925.html.
Shulman, Neil, M.D., et al. *Your Body's Red light Warning Signals: Medical
    Tips that May Save Your Life.* New York: Dell, 1999.
Shulman, Neil, M.D., James Reed, M.D., and Charlene Shucker. *The Black
    Man's Guide to Good Health.* Roscoe, IL: Hilton Publishing, 2001.

Chapter 22

Chopra, Deepak, M.D. *Quantum Healing: Exploring the Frontiers of
    Mind/Body Medicine.* New York: Bantam Books, 1990.
Cousins, Norman. *Anatomy of an Illness as Perceived by the Patient.* New
    York: Bantam, 1981.
Cousins, Norman. *Head First: The Biology of Hope and the Healing Power
    of the Human Spirit.* New York: Penguin, 1990.
Fiore, Neil, Ph.D. *The Road Back to Health: Coping with the Emotional
    Aspects of Cancer.* Berkeley, CA: Celestial Arts, 1990.
Lerner, Michael, Ph.D. *Choices in Healing: Integrating the Best of*

Conventional and Complementary Approaches to Cancer. Cambridge, MA: MIT Press, p.1114.

Siegel, Bernie S., M.D. *Love, Medicine, & Miracles: Lessons Learned About Self-Healing from a Surgeon's Experience with Exceptional Patients.* New York: Harper & Row, 1986.

Siegel, Bernie S., M.D. *Peace, Love, & Healing: Body/Mind Communication and the Path to Self-Healing.* New York: Harper & Row, 1989.

Chapter 24

Boston Women's Health Book Collective. *Our Bodies, Ourselves.* New York: 1998, pp. 579–581.

Caposella, Cappy, and Sheila Warnock. *Share the Care: How to Organize a Group to Care for Someone Who Is Seriously Ill.* New York: Fireside/Simon & Schuster, 1995.

Duda, Deborah. *A Guide to Dying at Home.* Santa Fe, NM: John Muir Publications, 1982.

Secundy, Marian Gray et al. *Trials, Tribulations, and Celebrations: African-American Perspectives on Health, Illness, Aging and Loss.* Yarmouth, ME: Interculturral Press, 1992.

GLOSSARY

adenoma: small, benign tumor

adjuvant therapy: chemotherapy and/or radiation given before or after surgery

advance medical directive: patient's wishes concerning medical treatment when the only possible outcome is death

alopecia: hair loss

anastomosis: joining of severed bowel

anemia: pathological deficiency of red blood cells

angiogram: x-ray of the blood vessels

antioxidants: nutrients that may help protect against cancer

aspiration: removal of fluid from a cyst or tumor with a syringe and needle

ascites: excess fluid in abdominal cavity

axilla: armpit

benign tumor: a lump or mass that is not cancer

biopsy: removal of a piece of tissue to see if it contains cancer

cancer: a term used for over one hundred diseases in which abnormal cells grow out of control

carcinoma: a cancer

carcinoma in situ: a cancer that has not spread

catheter: tube that allows for drainage of urine

cell: the basic structure of tissue or an organ

chemotherapy: chemical therapy

clinical trial: treatments that are part of a larger study to determine what treatments are most effective

colectomy: surgical resection of the bowel

colonoscopy: screening test for colon cancer

colostomy: surgical opening created for excretion purposes

cyst: a saclike structure in the tissue that contains fluid

duct: a tube through which body fluid passes

ductal carcinoma in situ (DCIS): abnormal cells that do not spread to underlying breast tissue but involve only the lining of a duct

endoscopy: screening test for diagnosing esophageal cancer

estrogen: a female hormone

etiology: causes of specific diseases

fecal occult blood test: a test for blood in the stool (feces)

gastroentrologist: stomach specialist

gynecologist: specialist in reproductive organs and diseases of women

hormones: chemicals produced by (endocrine) glands that then circulate in the body. Hormones go to other organs and affect their action.

hormone receptor test: test to measure amount of certain proteins (estrogen, progesterone) in tissue of the breast. Because hormones attach to these proteins, a high level of such hormone receptors probably means hormones are helping cancer grow.

hyperplasia: benign overproduction of cells

hysterectomy: surgical removal of part or all of the uterus

immune therapy: therapy that strengthens immune system

incontinence: inability to control urine

infiltrating cancer, invasive cancer, carcinoma: terms that describe a cancer that has spread beyond the tissue in which it formed

inflammatory breast cancer: describes condition in which cancer cells block the lymph vessels in the skin of the breast, causing the breast to become red, warm, and swollen—with the appearance of an infection.

lobe: a subdivision of an organ (breast, lung, etc.)

lobule: a subdivision of a lobe

lobular carcinoma in situ (LCIS): abnormal cells in the lobules of the breast. While LCIS seldom becomes frank cancer, it is a strong sign that a woman has increased risk of developing breast cancer.

lumpectomy: surgery that removes a cancerous breast lump and a rim of normal tissue around it

lymph: body fluid that travels through the lymph vessels. It carries cells that fight infection and cancer.

lymph nodes or **glands:** bead-shaped organs located along lymphatic vessels. They store the cells which trap and fight cancer cells and bacteria. Nodes are found in underarms, chest, neck, groin, and abdomen.

lymphedema: a swelling of the arm or leg from blocked lymphatics caused often by cancer, surgery, or x-ray treatment

lymphocytes: white blood cells

malignancyv cancer

mammogram: x-rays of the breast

mastectomy: surgical removal of breast

radical mastectomy: removal of breast, muscles of chest wall, and tissue under arm

modified mastectomy: same as radical except that muscles are not removed

mastistis: minor ailment that produces lumps

metastasis: spread of cancer beyond organ where cancer started

oncogenes: genes that cause tumors

oncologist: cancer specialist

otalaryngologist: ear, nose, and throat specialist

oxidants: irritants that may start growth of cancer cells

palliation: treatment that relieves symptoms (of cancer) but does not cure

Paget's Disease: cancer of breast producing rash on and about the nipple

palpation: process of examining an underlying organ by pressing
    on overlying skin

Pap smear: screening test to identify cervical cancer

pathology: the study of tissues and cells under the microscope

pathologist: doctor who does pathology

polyps: usually nonmalignant growth

progesterone: a female hormone

prognosis: likelihood of cure

prosthesis: replacement of part of the body with an artificial device

radiation (x-ray) therapy: treatment with high-energy rays to kill
    cancer cells

recurrence: reappearance of cancer after treatment has thought to
    have cured the disease

remission: signs and symptoms that cancer has disappeared.
    Remission may be temporary or permanent.

risk factor: anything that increases the chance of developing cancer

screening: tests or procedures to check for cancer or a disease
    when there are no symptoms

segmental mastectomy or **partial mastectomy:** removal of breast
    cancer by removing the tumor, surrounding tissue, and the
    covering over the underlying chest muscles. Some of the lymph
    nodes under the arm may also be removed.

sentinel lymph node biopsy: a dye or radioactive substance injected
    near the tumor that drains into nearest lymph node that cancer
    is likely to spread to. This lymph node once identified is
    removed.

stage: a system to identify how far the cancer has spread

subcutaneous: under the skin

systemic: reaching and affecting tissues and cells all over the body

tumor: an abnormal mass of tissue which may be benign or
    malignant

tumor marker: a substance obtained from blood or other body
    fluid that suggests the presence of cancer

urologist: surgeon specializing in urinary system

INDEX

acquired immunodeficiency syndrome. *See* HIV/AIDS

adenocarcinoma, 167, 221

adenoma (non-cancerous tumor), 47, 128

adjuvant therapy, 18–19, 58, 62

advance medical directive, 324

affirmations, healing benefits of, 299

African American men
and breast cancer, 274
and colorectal cancer, 82
and esophageal cancer, 192
most common forms of cancer, 13
and prostate cancer, 114–**115**, 116

African American women
and breast cancer, 13
and lung cancer, 110–111
most common forms of cancer, 13
reluctance to take part in clinical trials, 36, 44
and uterine cervical cancer, 154
and uterine endometrial cancer, 140–141, 148–149

African Americans
and cancer, 4–9, 13
and esophageal cancer, 192
and exercise, 285–286
having equal access to health care, 279–280
and HIV/AIDS, 250, 251
and justice in the health care system, 281
and kidney cancer, 186

Note: Page numbers in **bold** indicate a chart, table or illustration.
Index entries in CAPITALS indicate a major subject area covered in this book.